372662LV00003B/3/P
LVOW05s0419070214
Printed in the USA
CPSIA information can be obtained at www.ICGtesting.com

9 781457 517228

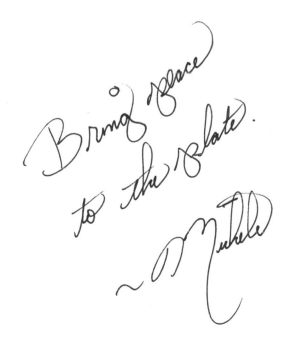

Bring peace
to the plate.

~ Michele

Praise for *No More Food Fights!*

"From acknowledging concerns and establishing shared values, to transparency and engagement, the topics addressed in Michele Payn-Knoper's *No More Food Fights!* offer a roadmap for today's ongoing national dialogue about food and farming. It all starts with listening and building trust and, at the end of the day, sharing personal stories rich in information so our customers can make informed decisions on their own and connect with farm and ranch families at the center of the plate."

—Bob Stallman, President, American Farm Bureau Federation

"Agriculture needs to address food buyer concerns in order to be successful in the future. Food buyers need to know more facts about where their food comes from. Michele Payn-Knoper bridges those worlds in *No More Food Fights!* and helps others do the same. A must-read."

—Mary Shelman, Harvard Business School Agribusiness Program

"There's no need to have food fights in the grocery aisles. *No More Food Fights!* provides a fresh look at some of the dilemmas food buyers and farmers both face. More importantly, this book gives ideas to get everyone around the food plate engaged in a conversation."

—Phil Lempert, The Supermarket Guru®, NBC News' Today Show Food Trends Editor, Author, and Speaker

"*No More Food Fights!* is a mantra everyone in agriculture should adopt. It's time to move beyond contentious, defensive rhetoric and engage in a conversation that recognizes that farmers and consumers alike want safe food produced responsibly. Use the insights offered by Michele Payn-Knoper to build your skills and enhance public understanding and appreciation of agriculture."

—Charlie Arnot, Center for Food Integrity

"There are many who know the need, but few who teach us how! In *No More Food Fights!*, Michele's valuable insight and examples teach others to bridge conversations from farm gate to consumer plate. Her years of living agriculture, leading connections, focused listening and targeted research combine to address vital needs for the creators and consumers of food. Read and internalize the message. Keep the book close by as a guide. Use the content. Meaningful conversations will be the result."

—Jolene Brown, Certified Speaking Professional,
Author of Sometimes You Need More Than a 2x4, and Iowa Farmer

"Canadian agriculturists need to pay close attention to the case studies in *No More Food Fights!*; these examples illustrate how people with limited connection to farming will impact our future. Michele Payn-Knoper provides common sense ways for people to connect around the plate. If you're interested in the future of food or farm, you need to read this."

—Shaun Haney, RealAgriculture.com

"*No More Food Fights!* takes a unique look at the very real problem of a disconnect between farm and food. Michele Payn-Knoper offers an intriguing look at tough issues such as food safety, animal welfare and biotechnology. We are delighted she brought food, nutrition and agriculture experts together."

—David Schmidt, President & CEO, International Food Information Council

"As a Canadian farmer, I was shocked to read that folks in downtown Toronto are actually afraid of their food! We produce great food for the world, and have close connections to where our food comes from, but that story is lost in translation. Michele's tips and insights will give all of us at the gate or the plate tools to make food conversations more helpful, and less fearful. Read *No More Food Fights!* to strengthen your advocacy for agriculture."

—Elaine Froese, Farm Family Coach, Seeds of Encouragement

NO MORE FOOD FIGHTS!

GROWING A PRODUCTIVE
FARM AND FOOD CONVERSATION

Food fights might seem entertaining, but there's nothing funny about the fights taking place over food production. Resource limitations, animal welfare, and biotechnology are just a few issues cropping up to create confusion in the grocery store. Ultimately, both farmers and food buyers are making a personal choice, and author Michele Payn-Knoper calls for decorum instead of mayhem in the conversation around farm and food.

In an effort to break stereotypes, one side of this book describes farmers who don't wear overalls but who do use technology in producing food and preserving the environment, dairy farmers who work on "cow comfort," and how hard farmers work on sustainability. On the other side, the book reminds farmers that only a tiny percentage of the population lives on a farm and urges farmers to tell their stories through social media and everyday conversation to correct mistaken beliefs about food production perpetuated by traditional media.

The book's very design lends itself to exploring both sides of the issue. One side of *No More Food Fights!* is aimed at those who primarily consume food—chefs, healthcare professionals, foodies, dietitians, and retailers. Flipping the book reveals the other side, which is geared toward those who produce food—farmers, agricultural businesses, and ranchers.

Throughout the book, the author intersperses personal stories from farmers, food scientists, dietitians, and ranchers. She naturally guides readers from both sides to "reach across the plate" to honestly explore food concerns and the critical connection from farm gate to food plate. Bring peace to your plate—and your next trip to the grocery store—with *No More Food Fights!* as your guide.

Sincere appreciation to the photography talent found throughout this book. Photo credits belong to the following individuals:
Food Chapters 3, 4, 6 and Farm Chapter 6: Joe Murphy
Food Chapter 5, Food & Farm Introductions and Farm Chapter 1, 7: Emmert Photography
Food Chapter 1, 7 and Farm Chapter 3: Lauren Chase, Montana Stockgrowers Association
Farm Chapter 2: Renee Kelly
Food Chapter 2: Zach and Anna Hunnicutt

Cover graphic by Kanaly Design

First published by Dog Ear Publishing
4010 W. 86th Street, Ste H
Indianapolis, IN 46268
www.dogearpublishing.net

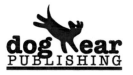

ISBN: 978-1-4575-1722-8

This book is printed on acid-free paper.

Printed in the United States of America

To my daughter, who serves as a daily inspiration to grow the conversation around food and farm. I hope you'll always love playing with cows and baking bread—and standing up for what you believe in.

Acknowledgements

"A life without cause is a life without effect."
~ Author unknown

Those words, on the wall above my desk, are a daily reminder of the power of serving a cause. An individual can't create effect without a community—I'd be remiss to not thank the many people my agricultural, food, and local communities.

More than 35 people from around the food plate contributed stories to this book and are recognized in the chapters, along with links so others can connect with these respected sources. I thank each person who allowed me to interview them, or provided their story in their own words. Your example added tremendous dimension to the discussion.

Talented photographers Joe Murphy, Lauren Chase of Montana Stockgrowers and Vicki Emmert graciously provided the beautiful photos at the beginning of each chapter. Thank you for bringing visual impact to *No More Food Fights!*

My office manager, Michelle Schrier, deserves appreciation for keeping my business moving along while I'm running around the world. You dealt with the wicked details of this book beautifully, which allowed me to think bigger.

Thank you to the clients across the United States and Canada who have entrusted me with "your people" for the last decade. You bring joy and meaning to my work, particularly when I see farmers reaching out and food buyers thinking differently as a result of our partnership.

I salute my professional speaker colleagues who helped inspire me to finally write this book, provide insight that the world outside of farming really doesn't understand haymows, and offer peer reviews. The same goes for the many advocates providing feedback and fodder.

Special appreciation to my closest girlfriends, who never know when their conversations with me will end up in a book or speech, but always support me. I treasure our friendship beyond words and am grateful for your perspective. I also respect your privacy enough to not share your real names with the world.

And last, but not least, thank you to my family who tolerates my driving passion for this work. My husband, who actually likes going to the grocery store, cares for our cattle and helps make it possible for me to do what I do. Our darling daughter, to whom this book is dedicated, is life's greatest blessing and a daily light in how important the cause of food and farming is to the future.

Table of Contents—Farm Side

No More Food Fights!

A Look at Agriculture's Future

"Who is responsible for the voice that will grow understanding between the farm gate and food plate?"

~MPK

When I look around a farm, the need for agriculture to tell our story becomes crystal clear. I walk into the barn and observe our cattle, which reminds me of how often farmers are portrayed as animal abusers. I want to bang my head against the barn wall as I think of the power of pictures and video in appealing to emotions.

Looking across the land, I reflect on people's angst about the types of products and practices used in the soil. I see large equipment filled with amazing technology and consider how some food buyers balk at technology in their food. I want to turn my back and just get back to work when I think of how polarizing the discussion has become.

But it's a group of giggling girls scampering through the pasture and playing in the haymow that leaves me firmly convinced of the need for each person in agriculture to do a better job of reaching a hand across the food plate. Yes, one of those girls is my daughter, who enthusiastically shares her love for dairy cattle with every friend who walks in the barn—a great reminder to all of us to do the same.

After all, that group of little girls will be buying food in 20 years. And they may be legislators, media, or neighbors determining the fate of how food should or should not be produced. In other words, they will influence your future.

Don't you want them to understand agriculture? If you're frustrated by today's misinformation about farming, the paperwork necessary to operate your business and media misinformation about agriculture—imagine the disconnect in 20 years. Who is responsible for the voice that will grow understanding between the farm gate and food plate?

Yesterday's practices won't rewrite tomorrow's history. Agriculture is not perfect; there are likely practices that need to be changed in farming and ranching. **One needed change is to hold agriculture accountable for having productive conversations to connect farm and food.**

After all, that conversation is happening with or without you—you decide whether your voice will be at the table. I consider it an honor to be a part of agriculture and feel each person has a responsibility to help determine agriculture's collective future. Do you?

What I believe:

1. Advocacy isn't about politics or public relations fluff. It's about creating—and growing—a movement through shared passions.

2. Food buyers deserve choice, just as farmers and ranchers deserve choice in how to operate.
3. If you wait to engage in the conversation until there's a problem, you're too late.
4. Firsthand experience is under-valued. People working with farm animals, registered dietitians, those caring for the soil and food scientists are experts who need to be telling their story.
5. Community is not about an individual, but is about individual contributions to a collective cause that's much bigger than one person. The leveraging factor of community multiplies impact and leverages an idea to become a movement.
6. Agriculture has failed in having a true conversation with food buyers in the past. We will lose our right to farm as we see fit if we make the same mistakes in the future.
7. True thought leadership is about looking at the big picture, having enough guts to try something new, engaging others in your cause and then getting out of the way.
8. Humans relate to humans; authenticity is simply sharing what you do and care about through conversation, Facebook, Twitter, telegraph, etc.
9. Science, research and economics will be met with deaf ears until you've connected through the heart. Yes, feelings matter!
10. United we stand, divided we fall. Those who condemn production practices different than their own damage the greater good of agriculture.
11. Social media isn't the answer to every communications problem, but it's a great way to immediately extend the reach of 1.5% of the population.
12. Farmers and the non-farm public can happily co-exist if you connect on shared values.

This book puts those principles into action. *No More Food Fights!* is the culmination of more than a decade of working to translate agriculture to the rest of the world. The book's emphasis is on you, your story, and how you can develop connections with people influencing your future.

You'll find 6 ½ steps designed to help folks in agriculture more effectively connect with people around the food plate. After all, food fights can be entertaining for a short time, but they get rather messy and smell bad when they've gone too far. Bystanders are hit with rotten tomatoes or fall down on the slimy floor. And the bullies who likely started the food fight slink away unnoticed, their pockets stuffed for another fight.

Is that really the scenario we want when we talk about food and farming? I think not. Is all the negativity and grandstanding really necessary? Frankly, I'm tired of the food fight and the drama around the issues. **How about we try to grow the food conversation with civility, seeking connections around the plate?**

Why? Because it's the right thing to do. Because it's important to find some understanding—an intersection of values—in the debate around farm and food. I invite you to join me in adding decorum—a big word for common courtesy—to the debate. My hope is that you'll give serious consideration that the discussion around food and farming should include civility.

If all you can think of right now is "Yes, but... (they don't understand, I need to educate people, etc.)." I suggest you put the book down and reconsider your intent. Just know that you're smelling up the place for the rest of us—and you'll eventually be throwing your rotten veggies at the mirror, so kindly take your fight to another room.

For the rest of you interested in exploring food and farm issues with responsibility and respect, join me in the journey. **Let's move the conversation about food and farming to a different level.** You'll find the stories of people from all around the food plate shared throughout this book to make it a richer discussion with more diverse perspectives.

What you put in your mouth is a personal choice. What a farmer produces is also a personal choice. One should not overpower the other.

I hope this side of the book will help people most closely connected with agriculture (farmers, agribusinesses, ranchers, ag organizations, et al.) find a framework for a more meaningful conversation with those on the food side. *No More Food Fights!* is designed help you build connections with the food side of the plate, engage in a civil discussion, and arm yourself with 6 ½ practical steps to tell your story.

It is time to engage in a conversation that reaches across the plate so we can celebrate choice. You'll know which side of the book you need to read based on your role around the plate; those with farm interests, start here. Those connected with the food side, flip over. You'll find an identical chapter in the middle focused on connecting at the center of the plate.

Who knows? You might be interested enough to read the other side when you're done. I challenge you to share the book with a person on the other side of the plate. My hope is that the ideas on each side will help grow a more productive conversation about farm and food.

My Farm Lens

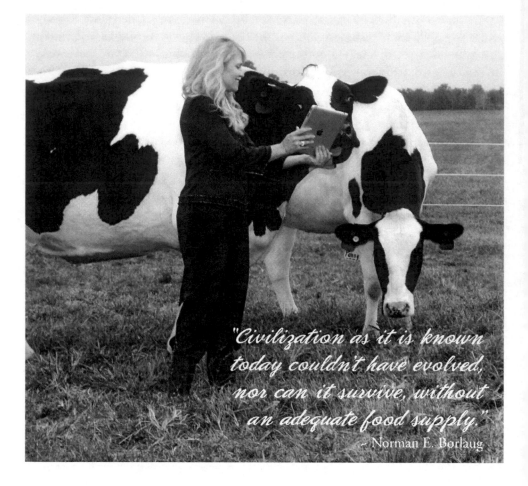

"Civilization as it is known today couldn't have evolved, nor can it survive, without an adequate food supply."
~ Norman E. Borlaug

Our family farm made me the person I am today. As a mom, I believe raising a family on a farm is the best upbringing you can give a child. I consider my work connecting the farm gate to food plate to be a calling. It is an honor to serve agriculture, and I am privileged to have spent my career doing that. You can get the full story at http://foodconvo.com/Qb8V0a.

Having said that, I want to be honest about some of the weaknesses in agriculture. Farmers are stubborn as mules and as independent as firecrackers streaking through dry grass. Modesty is interwoven into agriculture's fabric so tightly that it's uncomfortable talk about what we do. Agriculture is not always keen to ideas that come from "outsiders." Many farmers and ranchers become more than a little defensive when people ask questions. And agriculture is really good at preaching to the choir but not so hot at getting out into the pews.

I understand, as farmers and ranchers, you would rather be tending to your business, caring for your land or animals. Yet I also know that studies clearly show that people off the farm don't trust what you're doing. For example, Illinois Farm Families commissioned a study 2011 that reported **people still respect farmers but do not trust farmers' practices**. If you're like many in agriculture, this is a very personal issue—which means you feel attacked.

Many farmers have questioned why people don't trust the act of farming, but it's pretty simple to me: most Americans and Canadians are three to four generations removed from the farm. People living away from farms have little, if any, frame of reference for today's farming practices. In other words, they don't know what farming looks like until people show them pictures or videos or until they visit farms themselves.

Most (98.5%) of the US population does not live where farmers do. As such, they don't understand what you do. Do you really know how an automobile is built and what the latest technologies are to increase efficiency in those factories? Do you think about the people behind electricity when you flip a switch? Can you tell me how an iPhone or tablet is built?

Do you fully trust a practice or product if you don't understand it? Likely not, so let's be a bit more forgiving of people who don't know what happens on a farm. How are they supposed to know what you do in agriculture if you're not talking about it? Remember, people interested in where their food comes from is a good problem to have!

Agriculture is in the distinct minority, with only 1.5% of the population on a farm or ranch. The majority of US and Canadian citizens—those off the farm—are likely to determine how you will be able to operate if we continue to lose in the courtroom of public opinion.

According to a recent United States Farming and Ranching Alliance (USFRA) study, **72% of consumers know nothing or very little about farming.**[36] That screams opportunity for the majority of folks reading this!

What qualifies me to write this?

As we take a look at the 6 ½ steps of building connections, I'll do my best to represent many roles around the food plate. I've worked with farmers, food scientists, dietitians, foodies, ranchers, and chefs to gather their thoughts. You may not always like what you read, but *No More Food Fights!* has more than 50 stories representing diverse viewpoints and examples relevant to the farm side of the plate.

What qualifies me to write this book? I'm in the unique position of having a first-hand farm perspective and translating it to the non-farm public. I've been building communities to connect around the food plate in a variety of ways for 20 years. My love affair with food and farming started on a farm on southern Michigan, where I bought my first registered Holstein at nine years old. I'm thankful the view from my office still includes pretty black and white cattle on the small farm my husband and I built in west central Indiana.

Michigan State University provided my first glimpse of the marriage between farm and food as I went from dairy management to journalism to food science class while earning animal science and agriculture & natural resources communication degrees. It also gave me a taste of how damaging anti-agriculture activists can be.

My career has led me from working with farmers in more than 25 countries, to managing corporate relationships across 15 states for the National FFA Foundation, to building a speaking business to help people connect the farm gate to food plate to fork since 2001. I am honored to have received the Certified Speaking Professional designation, awarded to less than 10% of professional speakers globally.

I hope *No More Food Fights!* helps you think differently about the need to reach across the plate. I see a fork in the road between the farm gate and food plate—a divide that can be bridged through meaningful conversation. I don't believe that fork in the road has to be an 'either–or,' but should be a 'both.'

Won't you join me in growing connections across the plate?

6 ½ Steps to a
More Meaningful Conversation

"The most pathetic person in the world is someone who has sight but no vision."

~ Helen Keller

A mother has to return to work to cover legal costs. A dad who never had health issues now visits the doctor for stress-induced illness. A little girl so worried about her family farm being taken away that she has panic attacks. This is the reality of what activists do to family farmers. Count it as a wake-up call for any farmer who thinks it will never happen to their farm or ranch.

"Pray to God it doesn't happen to you" is the single message Alan Hudson wants his fellow farmers to know about his experience with activists. "Go to meetings even when it doesn't suit you and keep upon on the regulatory front." This poultry farmer from Maryland said it's not just about the hundreds of thousands of dollars in legal costs: it's the embarrassment of being in the local paper more than a kidnapper who murdered a little girl.

This extreme case, highlighted at http://foodconvo.com/12bkXco, is a wake-up call to anyone with a vested in agriculture. Are you frustrated by the lack of understanding about agriculture? Do you wish people would just leave you alone so you can get back to the business of farming? Are you tired by the constant insults and questions about food production?

Welcome to your new reality. Many people walk around the grocery store without a clue about who you are and what you do on a farm or ranch. Those that do don't necessarily trust farming practice. Others are heavily influenced by misinformation from activists.

Elected officials and state agencies have little perspective on the challenges of farming under intense regulations. The media seems to add to the onslaught with sensationalism from activist groups, and consumers readily admit they know very little about farming or ranching.

I understand your frustration. I also know your inbox is overflowing and chores are always waiting. But the reality is that we have to make time to connect around the food plate now because agriculture is losing in the courtroom of public opinion.

Whether you're an elevator manager, a seed salesman, or a farmer, *you* are the best person to have this conversation and to reach across the food plate because of your firsthand experience in agriculture.

Using the six questions as a starting point—who, what, why, when, where, how and you—put these steps into practice in starting a conversation with those on the other side of the food plate:

1. **Identify influencers.** Who can make a difference? Who are you the best at connecting with? Look at it the same way as you do hunting or playing a game of darts: you want to hit the bull's-eye.
2. **Find their hot buttons.** What's important to them? A hot button is an area of personal passion or pursuit—something that will really get them excited! Don't assume that you know; ask some questions to find out what they really care about.
3. **Translate agriculture to their hot buttons.** Don't data dump, but make a human connection through shared values.
4. **Invest 15 minutes daily.** Add "create a new food conversation" to your checklist. Consider it your opportunity to plant seeds for the future support of agriculture!
5. **Strategize where you can reach your target audience.** It may be at the county fair, at your grocery store, at the family dinner table, in your photos on Facebook, or simply in a discussion at church.
6. **Follow an action plan to develop long-lasting relationships.** Let it serve as your recipe for a healthy conversation about food and farm.
6 ½. **Put your passion to work!** You are the key ingredient.

Helping people understand agriculture doesn't have to be complicated. If you don't make a point to start investing 15 minutes today, what will you be harvesting in a year? 🦃

CHAPTER 1
Who? Know Your People

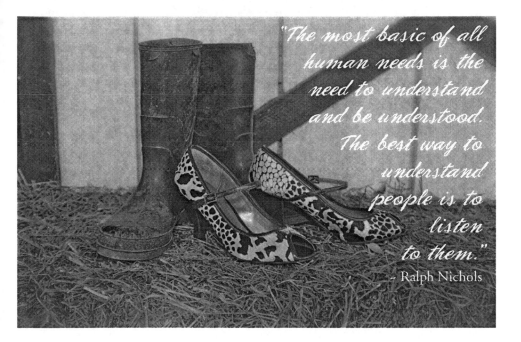

"The most basic of all human needs is the need to understand and be understood. The best way to understand people is to listen to them."
— Ralph Nichols

Everyone just needs to understand agriculture. Right? Wrong. If you approach this from strictly an educational standpoint, you're going to turn people away. After all, there's plenty of information floating around, lots of science, and centuries of research. **What we lack is the human connection.**

Instead, let's look at this as an opportunity to have a conversation about your experience in agriculture. A conversation that might lead to a human connection between farm and food. A conversation that doesn't involve screaming at each other or echoing across the food plate.

Finding the right people to connect with is a critical first step in the process, but do a quick mirror check first. Are people glad to know you? Glenna Salsbury's four principles of "making people glad they saw you" apply.[37]

1.   Be interested in others. Ask questions and listen to the answers.
2.   Be willing to display enthusiastic support for others.
3.   Find ways to rekindle individual enthusiasm for life and work.
4.   Help people expand their horizons for what *might be* instead of what *is*.

This doesn't mean you have to put on a show or always be in a good mood. Note that three of the four points revolve around others. This starts with knowing who you're likely to be the most comfortable having a conversation with. Then spend some thinking about different types of influencers. Finally, **realize it may be as difficult for you to understand their lives as it is for them to know what you're doing in agriculture.**

Great shoes and silage bags

Polka dotted. Zebra print. Fuscia platforms. Great shoes make a statement. They can be an opportunity to connect on a more human level. Really! They also teach a lesson about connecting with someone different from you.

How would you feel about trading a pair of size-12 work boots with size-6 floral wedges? Likely, a little awkward. Depending on which side you started on, you likely either have your nose curled up at dirty, smelly work boots or your toes crunched up in shoes half your size.

I'd like to introduce you my friend Eileen, the owner of those size-6 floral wedges. She lives in Fayetteville, Georgia, with her husband and four children. This upscale suburb is filled with great shops and restaurants—and many opinions about how you should be growing food.

A pretty little blonde, Eileen is originally from rural Indiana and lived on a small farm with both parents working as teachers. She was a cheerleader in high school, still evidenced in her big smile and fun personality. Eileen is now the stay-at-home mom of four kids under eight years old.

She's my window into the well-to-do suburban mom crowd, though her personal perspective on farmers is clearly tempered by her rural upbringing. Eileen tells me that she has friends who buy "hormone free" meat and milk. Some buy almond or soy milk to avoid hormones (yes, she knows all food has hormones in it). Other of her friends will only buy organic from Whole Foods so their kids are supposedly not exposed to pesticides. Some buy cage-free chicken and eggs because of animal cruelty concerns. Some of the questions these moms are asking:

> **CONNECTION POINT 1**
> More than 2/3 of those purchasing food are thinking about how it's produced on a regular basis. Consumers are looking for information about farming. All of us in agriculture have to determine if we're willing to give it to them — even during planting season, winter, harvest, or summer heat stress.

- Is my little girl going to develop earlier because of hormones in food?
- Why have farms gotten so big? They're like factories.
- Why shouldn't I avoid high fructose corn syrup? I don't want my kids to have that!
- Is meat bad?
- Why can't all farms be small and cute like the one we rent for our birthday parties?

These are intelligent women, most of whom have college educations. Eileen sometimes questions them about where they get their information. The most common sources are Dr. Oz, shows like *Ellen* (who is a great Wayne Pacelle fan), *Dr. Phil*, and what they read online. Very rarely, if ever, is a farmer mentioned.

Eileen's kids spend most of their time in the barn when they visit us in Indiana; they often can be found on the halter of our heifers and cows. We took them to our neighbor's milking parlor on their last visit so they could see milk produced firsthand. It was Eileen's comment outside of the parlor that left me thinking the most.

We were showing the kids the different feeds the cows ate over by the silage bags, letting the kids feel the feed and smell the fermented corn and hay, while explaining why dairy cattle need both to be healthy. Eileen paused by the bags, saying, "I always wondered what those white tubes were when we drove by."

It was a bit of a wake-up call to hear her say that; I realized how much we took for granted that people know about farms. After all, this was someone with knowledge of artificial insemination and calving and familiarity with crops. Yet the plastic bags that fermented feed had been a question mark for Eileen.

This reminded me to not only to do a better job in talking about the basics, but also that **people on the "inside" need to step back and look around agriculture.** What are the things you're doing differently than a generation or two ago—and why? That's likely what many questions are about.

People aren't ignorant or lazy just because they don't wear work boots every day. They simply haven't been around a farm to see all the changes and don't trust farming practices until someone explains it to them. Frankly, people in agriculture have not done a very good job of that.

Most likely, the majority of people even trust you as a farmer, so please don't be annoyed or defensive when they ask you questions. Realize that you may be just as ignorant about life in floral wedges as they are about life in work boots—and that **both sides can learn from each other.**

Jump out of the choir loft!

Consider who you really need to connect with if you're going to have a productive, meaningful conversation about agriculture. If it's a group of people who wear the same kind of shoes, think like you, and do what you do—it is time for you to go beyond the choir.

Stretch a bit and think about the type of people you'd like to approach as you jump out of the choir loft.

- Identify specific groups.
- Look for key influencers.
- Determine which groups you can be the most effective with.
- Write them down!
- Understand that you can change groups.

You may think you're too busy, but please understand that these influencers are being engaged— daily—by those who are speaking for farmers. The Humane Society of the United States (HSUS), Greenpeace, People for the Ethical Treatment of Animals (PETA) and other activist groups are talking about what you do—and they are becoming known as experts.

Experience with farm groups across the world tells me you're not likely to be comfortable with being thrust into the spotlight. **Start small. Focus on where you can make an impact—and then grow your efforts.**

A shy "old" farmer on national media

A great example of doing just that is Larry Sailer from Iowa. Larry is like many who have farmed for decades; he has ridden the highs and lows through vast changes.

One of the ways he has responded is to leave the safety of his farm and identify different influencer groups that he could engage in conversation. **It was not natural or comfortable for him, but it has helped farmers have a voice.** His story clearly illustrates ways to work with different influencers; he's moved from presenting to local civic groups to talking with elected officials to hosting international media on his farm.

I started farming in the great farming times of the 1970s. It was very difficult at that time to do wrong. Exports were exploding and prices were good. New technology was helping to control weeds and increase our yields. Little did I know, this was setting me up for a tough fall.

Our communication at the time was very primitive. AM radio, three channels on the TV, and our phone was a party line shared by three farm families and a business. Few words were being added to our communication. I'm not sure cell phones or the internet were even a dream.

Along came the '80s. Farming had become the game of extremely conservative farmers that did not over expand and kept some money in reserve. This is when I discovered you don't do it on your own. Outside forces have a huge impact on my farm operation.

Government intervention, beginning with the grain embargo, completely changed the playing field. I knew it was time to get off the sanctity of my farm and leave behind the security blanket of hard work to get involved. I wanted to influence people that I saw having a huge impact on farming and ranching. Government regulation and policies were becoming as much a part of farming as doing chores.

For the next 25 years, I worked with farm organizations such as Farm Bureau and Iowa Pork Producers, trying to give farmers a voice at the table. Even though I've always been an extreme introvert and shy farm boy, I started giving speeches to civic groups for the National Pork Board.

I learned a lot talking to the generations of folks who moved from the farm to cities. Being removed from the farm, it did not occur to them that farming could change. And the kids that grew up without any connection to the farm think that their food is made at the grocery store.

When I talked to civic groups, I would normally have 15 to 30 people to share my story with. One time I had a crowd of 175 in Ames, Iowa. This old farm boy really was thinking he should be home doing chores! Much to my delight, this young urban group proved to be the best audience ever. Before I spoke, they sang a song one of them had written in my honor about hog farming, which pretty well cemented my attachment to sharing what I do and why I do it.

My favorite part of these talks is the question-and-answer segment at the end. This is the part where I get to learn. A conversation must include listening. I'm not out there to preach about my perceptions about what is right. I'm there to listen and learn. I need to know the concerns of people and to learn how they view what I do. I don't live on old McDonald's farm anymore, and my farm animals are not the same as the cartoon characters you see on TV.

ROTTEN VEGETABLE 1
Some people consider agricultural advocacy as public relations fluff. Ron Bailey, in book The Law of Fear Mongering, pointed out that it costs $10 to refute every $1 invested by the fear mongers.
The reality of today's agrifood business is that we are seeing bottom-line impact from the misinformation about our industry, an impact that's likely to increase significantly if we don't make some changes.

Larry did a great job of starting where he felt the most comfortable and then growing his comfort zone. You'll hear more from him in Chapter 6.

Prioritize influencer groups you feel most comfortable starting with. Once you clearly understand who you're trying to connect with, you'll be able to identify what their hot buttons are.

What's important to them? This hot button is different for each person and can be about quality of life, family, socioeconomic status, safety, or profitability. If you can appeal to these hot buttons for your influencer group, you're going to be able to translate agriculture to their language. More on that in the next two chapters!

Who is going to influence your future?

Consider how these influencer groups present an opportunity for you to engage in meaningful conversation. Which will influence your future the most? Who are you most comfortable beginning with? Is there another group that represents a long-term goal for you?

CONNECTION POINT 2
How is your promise-to-delivery ratio? Do people always know that you're going to deliver what you say you will? Every time you tell somebody you're going to follow up, treat it as a promise. It doesn't matter if you use a smartphone, planner, Post-It notes, or notes on your arm—make sure your promise-to-delivery ratio is 110%.

Media	Medical professionals
Teachers	Chefs
Restaurants	Extension educators
Parents	Food processors
Celebrities	Religious organizations
Diet & fitness industry	Researchers
Doctors	Community leaders
Consumer groups	Farmers
Dietitians	Government agencies
Food retailers	Post-secondary educators
Land owners	Elected representatives
School administrators	Farm organizations
Elementary students	Baby boomers
High school students	Nurses
College students	Moms
Preschools	Dads
Extended family	Food writers/journalists
Neighbors	Food service
Friends	Health and lifestyle programs
Government	Personal trainers
Retailers	Politicians
Agribusiness	Civic or service groups

Are you remembered as a person who cares?

The first step in building a relationship is creating rapport. Your goal should be to establish an atmosphere of trust and respect. It's not just about telling your story, it's about getting to know somebody. How do you do this?

- Do your homework. If you were referred, ask the referrer about the person you're going to meet with. If not, do some research online.
- Know the power of a person's name. Remember the person's name, use it frequently, and, if it's a tricky one, confirm that you're pronouncing it correctly.
- Be respectful of the person's time. If you have a scheduled time to meet or talk and the other person sounds rushed or constantly checks his or her watch, ask if it's a bad time and reschedule.
- Look for signs. An office (or a Facebook wall) is a looking glass into a personality type. Ask questions about the person's family if you see photos, talk about his or her hobby if the decor makes the favorite pastimes obvious, or ask about the awards you see prominently displayed. A straightforward personality with a more stark office will want to get directly to business, so be ready to discuss industry trends and ask for insight.
- Show your personality. People connect with people. Don't be as stiff as a board, especially if you're uncomfortable. Let them see what you're made of!

- Listen with genuine concern. This person is meeting with you because he or she has a problem or need. Don't offer advice at this stage; just listen and show empathy.

Why is building rapport important? It's the first step to show that you're sincerely interested in a mutually beneficial relationship. **Take the time to learn something about the person you're trying to connect with. You will be remembered as a person who cares.**

If it's to be, it's up to me

A great case study on targeting a group of influencers and building rapport is Debbie Lyons-Blythe, a cattle rancher in the Flint Hills of Kansas. She and her husband raise 500 head of cattle and have five children—two in high school and three in college. Debbie is one of those women who do it all and put others at ease with a smile. She's naturally outgoing but doesn't have a lot of free time between raising her family, running the ranch, and participating in several leadership roles.

Her husband's family homesteaded their farm in 1890 and Debbie and her husband are proud to continue the heritage of ranching and conserving the land. Debbie didn't have time for this "advocacy stuff" until she realized how the lack of understanding about agriculture was going to affect their business and family. As a result, she started blogging at kansascattleranch.blogspot.com and has made media appearances such as *Anderson Cooper Live.*

CONNECTION POINT 3
Hot buttons may or may not be related to ag, farming, or food; don't expect them to be. Not everyone worries about food and farm issues 24 hours a day; they have many other interests.

We've all heard the numbers that less than 2% of the population is involved in agriculture. We've all read the headlines about GMOs Unsafe, Farmer Charged with Animal Cruelty. And, we've all thought that someone should straighten out the facts and get the story straight.

You've likely heard "If it's to be, it's up to me." This is the foundation of agricultural advocacy. Every farmer and rancher wants to combat the misinformation and tell the truth about agriculture. But the nature of the job is that farmers and ranchers are busy! We work 7 days a week, 365 days a year and sometimes more than 12 hour days. Who has time for agvocacy?

"If it's to be, it's up to me." Two years ago, my husband's second cousin brought her young family to visit us on the ranch for a week. She will one day be part owner in some land that we manage, due to the foresight of her great grandfather. He left the land in trust to his grandchildren. Today only one of the six grandchildren is actively involved in agriculture—my husband. This gal only visits the farm that her ancestors homesteaded; she brings her family "to the farm" for a vacation infrequently. Her roots are in this land and with the cattle on it, but she has no first-hand knowledge of what I do here every day.

Her questions about the safety of the beef and milk that we fed our families during their visit were the impetus for me to begin my blog. Like so many ranchers, I knew I needed to reach out to consumers to let them see how I raise cattle, but I couldn't justify the time spent on something so frivolous as writing a blog or tweeting a photo from the tractor seat. But the same day her family left to return to their Denver home, I began to write about my life on a Kansas ranch.

I chose the title "Life on a Kansas Cattle Ranch" because that is exactly what I decided to write about. I began with, "I'm a wife, a mother to five teenagers and a cattle rancher." I often remind people that I am no one special. I am just a cattle rancher, who happens to be a woman, and I love to write. So I have chosen that avenue to spread the word about how cattle are raised. I am only special because I have consciously chosen to spend time advocating for agriculture every day.

I target "Moms who live in the city." I chose that group because I feel that as a mom, I can relate to them very well. We have the same concerns, questions and stressors. I spend more time connecting with my target audience than I do writing my blog post. As a journalist, writing is easy for me.

But just as important as a well-written blog post, is having someone to read it! I use Twitter and Facebook, as well as Pinterest and YouTube to connect with other moms. I tweet about my kids' ball games, their successes at school and our failures and challenges as a family. I give, and receive, advice from moms active on social media—keeping in mind that creating and maintaining a relationship is all about making a connection. I can then share my link to my blog with people who I know will read it and share it around as well.

Specific outcomes have been the relationships I have created and friendships I value. I am not about having the highest numbers or ranking on Klout—what matters to me are the conversations and opportunities for swapping information. I aim for quality, not quantity. I aim for valuable conversations each week, instead of a certain number of page views. Talking among ourselves (other ag advocates) is fun and sometimes helpful, but I don't have much time to spend "goofing off" with them. I use my time on social media to converse with my target audience, and any other conversations are just icing on the cake!

> **ROTTEN VEGETABLE 2**
> You may think that feeding a growing population is important to everyone around the food plate, but it's a much higher priority to farmers and ranchers. Only 25% of consumers believe they have a responsibility in that, according to the Center for Food Integrity.

There are some great agvocates out there telling our story. But we need more! There are so many activists and wing nuts with the goal to put farmers and ranchers out of business—we must get the facts and the truth out there! If you have any interest in agvocating, do not put it off because you are too busy, or you don't know how to start a blog. Don't let Twitter or Facebook scare you! Jump in and give it a try.

Investing 15 minutes a day in your future

Invest 15 minutes a day to tell your story about what you do on your farm or ranch. Be yourself; don't worry about trying to be perfect. The people who want to know would like to see that we are human and we care about what we are doing.

Don't wait. Start small, and you can build from there. Take 15 minutes to post a Facebook status that mentions agriculture…then when you have time, start a blog or open a Twitter account. Connect with consumers wherever you can—they are hungry for information!

If you want to see how targeting specific groups of influencers pays off, check out the comments and questions from all sorts of moms on Debbie's blog. That's what going beyond the choir looks like—she invested the time to do something that wasn't natural and knew exactly who she was focused on.

Selecting which group you're comfortable talking to is crucial to ensuring your success. There are as many influencer groups to choose from a there are seed varieties. You determine which influencer group is the best for your field and then begin planting the seeds. You adapt according to changing conditions. It's important you spend time selecting the right influencer group and tend to it in your personal action plan to make the harvest you desire.

CHAPTER 2

What? Find Their Hot Buttons

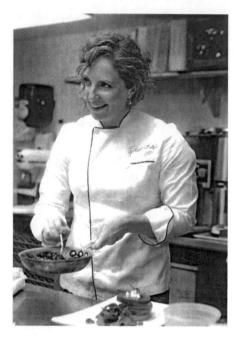

"It takes a great person to be a good listener."

~Calvin Coolidge

A simple way to quickly move a conversation to a different level is to think in terms of others. Dale Carnegie has said the most magical thing to another person is his or her own name; my philosophy is that finding and hitting a person's hot button runs a very close second. A hot button is a need or interest area, something a person feels passionate about.

A hot button is a priority to that person or a potential, a need to be addressed if you want to connect your cause. A hot button can be positive or negative. What are the hot buttons for the groups you're likely to talk to? Think about the people you identified in your conversation clusters.

Consider this: you're selling a car. Your customer's true need is transportation. The need is mixed with the hot buttons of safety, image, speed, and more. The priority of the hot buttons will change by age group, social class, and the economy. The final buying decision will likely be made on priority hot buttons.

Just ask questions

How do you identify a hot button for the influencer group you're targeting? Preliminary research will give you some indication, but **the best way to find a hot button is to simply *ask* and then *listen*!** Asking questions is critical to successfully connecting your cause, plus it will help you feel more knowledgeable and less likely to be rejected.

Asking questions doesn't have to be complicated or even intrusive; it's merely an opportunity to learn more about the person or group you're talking to. If you're stumped about what to ask, think about the six elements of a story—who, what, why, where, when, and how.

Once you start asking questions, you'll quickly make the other person feel at ease because you're showing interest in him or her and it will become easier for you to understand the person's hot buttons. This will also help address the potential concern about not being able to relate to non-ag people—as you learn more about them, you'll understand their values.

Shared values are three to five times more important in building trust than is demonstrating competence, according to a nationwide study conducted by the Center for Food Integrity.[38] In other words, the person you're conversing with isn't likely to be interested in your farming practices until you connect to each other as humans. That's why learning about the other person is so important.

Many farmers and ranchers define themselves by what they do, which can make human connection more difficult. Consider what interests and values you have outside of farming. Those are where you find shared values with the non-farm public. Shared values build trust, which then—and only then—gives you permission to talk about what you do.

Chef understands where you're coming from

One of the groups around the food plate that remains a mystery to the majority is restaurants and chefs. Don't get me wrong—my husband and I enjoy special restaurants a great deal and have been known to drive long distances for the right kind of chef, but there's a mystique in the chasm between many farmers and the restaurant side of the plate.

It's likely been propagated by campaigns such as Chipotle's 2012 Super Bowl ad[39] and furthered by several major chains falling prey to HSUS's pressure tactics. And, if you're like us, you're more than a little disgusted by

---

CONNECTION POINT 4

How do you identify a person's hot buttons? It's actually quite simple... ask questions! Spend some time with your target to ask some open—ended questions. Listen to what that person shave to say and then ask a few more follow—up questions about the ideas the person seems to really care about. Remember, listening is your number—one skill in a conversation. The second most important skill? Observing! Look at the person you're talking with and see what you can learn from their tone, space (office, Facebook wall, photos), and reactions

the responses you usually get from wait staff when you inquire about the origins of the food in a restaurant or exactly what the restaurant's "natural" label means.

Conversations with chefs and restaurant owners are a window into a portion of the food plate that agriculture needs to understand, however. I recently had the opportunity to spend time with chef and restaurateur Renee Kelly. She's a fiery red-head who has created a dining experience in a castle in the Kansas City, Kansas, area. She recently transitioned the beautiful restaurant Renee Kelly's Harvest to a farm-to-table concept using local and regional farmers. You can see it for yourself at http://www.reneekellys.com/.

Renee loves the idea of buying from her neighbor, but she balances that with an understanding of feeding a hungry population. "Treat your food with respect and treat the environment with respect, it will come back to you" is her mantra. We had a very lively conversation about her food interests as a restaurateur. I asked her a few questions and then listened to her talk, while managing not to argue or dissect her answers (my tongue bears the scars to prove this).

When I inquired what a productive conversation between a commodity farmer and customer might look like, she immediately turned to asking questions. She also hopes the customer would ask the farmer many questions:

- *What do you do?*
- *What does your day/quarter look like?*
- *When do you have to plan?*
- *How many chemicals do you need to use?*
- *What are the insects?*
- *Can you share your trials and tribulations of the seasons?*
- *Once your food is harvested, where does it go?*
- *Do you know how many people you help feed?*
- *Do you take pride in what you do? To what degree?*
- *Do you have your kids help you, farm with multiple generations?*
- *How did you get started?*
- *Why did you choose to grow what you're growing and how you're growing it?*
- *Are you willing to share your daily expenses?*
- *Can you tell me about subsidized crops from a farmer's perspective?*

Renee simply **asks for the farmer to be open-minded, willing to talk, and patient enough to explain what he or she does, without getting offended: "Give us a simplified kindergarten explanation."** She mentioned that she uses "I understand where you're coming from" frequently to soften the tone of the conversation.

In nearly the same breath, Renee wished for a fact-based conversation and acknowledged that she's never had a conversation about food without emotion. She wants to talk about the "softer side of business" to move the conversation from point A to point B: "Give me *Reader's Digest* verbiage."

It was clear that Renee is a storyteller herself, so it didn't surprise me that **she asked for farmers and agriculture to tell better stories** (of the nonfiction variety, of course). "I understand farmers are not the type to scream from the mountaintop," she said, but she clearly wants agriculture to make farming real through stories: "It's very important farmers communicate their story—what they do and where they come from." Renee suggested stories that she can retell in her restaurant or that other influencers can retell. She also pointed to the need for the chef, butcher, grocery store, and wait staff to understand the stories.

She asked several times for a start-to-finish description. Growing season to harvest. What happens when grain or animal leaves your farm? We keep hearing about transparency and wondering exactly what it is—I suspect the answer lies in our ability to tell the start-to-finish story.

Renee understands that chemicals need to be used in farming, but she'd like to know specifically why and how farmers got to the place where they use the chemicals on the farm. She also believes animals are treated well on farms and that videos illustrating animal cruelty are of bad apples who give farmers a bad name—and increase media ratings.

She does have concerns about large animal operations and wants animals to be raised in the manner in which they were meant to be. When I probed further about the concerns with large farms, she used teacher-student ratio as an example: "In a classroom with 15 kids, you are a better teacher and give students individual attention. If that's tripled, you can't possibly give the same attention to each child. That doesn't mean the teacher suddenly becomes a horrible teacher or a bad person. The same is true for farms." Yet, she's thrilled with the progress in animal care that allows her to cook pork to only 145 degrees and serve a more tender dish to her customers.

Renee encourages farmers and ranchers to keep an open mind in these conversations but knows that's especially difficult when it's your livelihood. She used her own example to drive home how "when you cook your specialty and someone tells you it's done wrong, it's hard to swallow. I know it's difficult for farmers to swallow what people are saying when the person has never been on a farm."

"Awesome people who grow food" was her quick answer when I asked about what came to mind when she thinks about farmers. "I think about the big guy and the little guy." She is more likely to communicate with small farmers and views them as more apt to invite her to their farms to see what's going on and also feels they're more likely to pay attention to what they grow. "They work it every day, unlike the large commodity growers."

As a buyer, Renee has found that small farmers love to talk about food and ask her what she needs. They want to know what customers are looking for and what differences she hears about from customers (e.g., when feed is changed in the chickens' diet) and are excited to have the conversation. She finds a lot of gaps in the type of farming and types of communications they have with customers.

"People are fascinated by farms but far removed with where their food comes from. They can't identify with farmers because food is so readily available that customers just assume it's easy to farm." The need for a conversation around the plate is evident when you couple that misconception with how consumers know they're supposed to be eating better but don't know what that means.

Chef Renee's most easily identifiable hot button? Know your food and where it's grown, as she believes food equals health. And she knows farmers have a very big responsibility in that. She also knows that others, such as servers and chefs, will substantially influence her customers' perceptions of the food.

Forging human connections through questions

How can you develop a relationship or connection with someone who has such different interests than yours, like chefs and restaurant servers? The secret is in identifying their needs and hot buttons. It wasn't difficult to get Chef Renee to talk in our interview—I simply asked questions and recorded her answers, listening carefully for excitement that indicated a hot button.

Meaningful conversations begin with focus on the other person. Invest time in these techniques to uncover hot buttons:

- Ask open-ended questions to learn more about a person's interests, whether related to agriculture or not.
- Realize that even the most driven businessperson or outspoken adversary is a human being and has very human interests.
- Observe body language and subtle signs that indicate a person's hot button, such as eyes lighting up, eyebrows raising, or enthusiasm on social media.
- Look around the person's space for items of interest, such as office décor, awards, photos, interest shared in social channels, etc.
- Continue to ask questions.
- Make note of areas you can ask the person to elaborate on and reconfirm the hot buttons you've heard.
- Listen to what the person has to say, and then ask a few more follow-up questions about the ideas he or she seems to really care about. Remember, listening is your best way to connect.
- Understand that you do not have to agree with the other person's hot buttons.

As you are listening to others, I would encourage you to ask yourself how open agriculture is to sharing information from all sides of the food plate. Are we clear about the roles of scientists in monitoring and improving food? Do we effectively explain the technology used to improve food and nutrition? Do farmers fully appreciate what others around the food plate contribute? I think not.

Science, accuracy, and credibility are hot buttons shared by food producers, dietitians, and scientists. The frustration with food trends, misinformed celebrity "experts," and the inability to connect facts are other common needs, but I rarely see the connection across our food plate happening between these groups.

Let's take a look at dietitians as another example. Many times when I'm training agricultural audiences to speak out, people will mention RD's "tell you what to not eat" when I ask what they know about dietitians. Folks in agriculture really need to know more about this group of influencers, given our obesity epidemic, aging baby boomer population, and increasing interest in nutrition.

Are farmers the only ones making food?

The great news is that farmers and registered dietitians share several key hot buttons. Don't take my word for it; Marianne Smith Edge, MS, RD, LD, FADA, is Senior Vice President, Nutrition & Food Safety, for the International Food Information Council (IFIC). She brings 25 years of experience to the table from the food business—and happens to have a firsthand farm perspective.

As someone who grew up on a family-owned dairy farm in Kentucky, I was immersed in daily activities and chores that some people would consider less than glamorous. However, little did I know, I was laying the foundation for a career in food, nutrition, and agriculture. As a registered dietitian with a background in farming, and a current farm owner, I have a unique perspective on the real world of food and nutrition.

We often hear the phrase "farm to fork" used to describe the process our food undergoes to reach our dinner plates. I argue that we sometimes use the phrase far too casually. Our food production system includes farmers, food manufacturers, distributors, grocers, food-service establishments, and others. It takes all of these roles to bring us a variety of safe, high-quality foods that are also tasty, convenient, nutritious, fresh, and affordable. Yet, in many instances, there is a disconnect among this process and the consumer.

It is important to my job as a registered dietitian and communicator to help bridge the gap between the different entities involved in the food continuum. To help expand my career in the field of food, health, and nutrition, I joined the International Food Information Council Foundation to help further its mission to effectively communicate science-based information on health, nutrition, and food safety for the public good. Science and technology are essential components to understanding the complexity of food.

There is no simple answer establishing meaningful conversations, but the core communication principles I follow and encourage others to consider include listening, learning, and engaging.

It is important to remember that we cannot communicate in silos but we must keep everyone involved, particularly the consumer. It is easy to make assumptions and presume food buyers are informed, but that simply is not always the case as fewer and fewer consumers have a direct link to your work as a farmer. We should seek to understand consumer needs and answer their questions—and they have questions. Research is one opportunity to gain consumer insights, and another is to simply listen.

Consumers have a growing interest about their food. They have an interest in wanting to know what is in their food and why. Explaining agriculture, modern food technology, and food processing may not always result in a harmonious discussion.

Terms such as "fresh," "whole," "organic," and "natural" foods often evoke emotion and convey such positive overtones. However, I contend that these terms, in addition to processing, and technology, can coexist. Both fresh and processed foods can be safe, nutritious, and environmentally responsible choices.

I acknowledge that there will be disagreements about food, generally, but we need more conversations where we can meet in the middle and find common ground. Ultimately, it is about our ability to continue to have the abundance of safe, affordable, and nutritious food to which we have been accustomed.

Agriculture has and will continue to make advancements like all other areas of our lives—we ultimately demand it. But society demands advancements to be made in a responsible and sustainable manner—a focus for which we all need to participate.

As a registered dietitian, communicator, and "farm girl," I contend that we can and will benefit from expanding the scope of our conversations to broaden our understanding! Real advancement will occur when we realize working together will provide the benefits for which we all strive—improving and maintaining the overall health of society.

Interesting opportunity for agriculture, don't you think? The more you work with influencers on the food side, the more opportunities you'll discover. Marianne is a past president of the American Dietetic Association (ADA), now the Academy of Nutrition and Dietetics (AND). You'll find IFIC referenced throughout *No More Food Fights!* It is one of my favorite sources as a nonprofit organization that effectively communicates sound, science-based information on nutrition and food safety.

Are we taking care of hungry people at home?

We spend a lot of time in agriculture talking about feeding a population expected to double by 2050. Interestingly enough, feeding the world only resonates with 25% of Americans,[40] but food insecurity within the US draws a great deal more compassion.

Have you ever lived in hunger? Have you worked with or helped those in need of food? Have you asked them what's important to them? If not, it's a great opportunity to ask questions and relate to others' concern about rising food prices. A 10% increase in food prices would make life unbearable to many, so their chief concern isn't about labels—it's about economical food.

Contrary to common belief, you won't find many people who are on food stamps long term. As it turns out, people living in food insecurity don't like to be judged by a few rotten apples who perpetuate that impression any more than farmers like having manure thrown all over their image by sensationalized videos.

Paul McConaughy from Michigan Nutrition Network (find him on Twitter at @MiNutrition) pointed to four myths about people who need help with food:

ROTTEN VEGETABLE 3
Citing only research and statistics when trying to connect with consumers isn't a good idea. Sure, science-based information is important to share, but not until you connect on an emotional level. A sociology study from Iowa State University found that "communicating only facts to consumers is a recipe for failure..." Let's not keeping making the same mistake.

- It's their fault...if only they managed better.
- They're not my neighbors.
- They aren't really hungry...they're abusing the system.
- People who are hungry are "chronically" poor...they stay on benefits forever.

Paul provided background on those needing food assistance, their concerns, and what this largely unseen portion of the food plate looks like:

"Tell people they are better than they think they are and they'll do better than they think they can do," said Rev Julian DeShasier, Senior Minister, University Church Chicago in the movie The Line.

In 2011, one in seven Americans—46 million people—received supplemental nutrition assistance (SNAP), the new name for food stamps. The average amount they received was $134 per person each month. Twenty-five percent of American children receive SNAP.[41]

People needing food assistance live in every community and come from every walk of life. Despite the assumption that the hungry are chronically poor, half of all new SNAP recipients received benefits for 10 months or less. Seventy-four percent of new participants left the program within two years. They may come back, because working your way out of poverty isn't easy, but they aren't getting on SNAP and staying. Over forty percent of recipients are working. The average American family spends seven percent of their income on food. Those in poverty spend as much as thirty percent.[42]

How do people get to be in need of food? The two most common reasons are financial or medical emergencies. Financial emergencies could be caused by natural disasters like Hurricane Katrina, or by the sudden collapse of the financial markets. For many people it could be the loss of a job or sometimes even a reduction of scheduled work hours. Medical emergencies include the need for high cost care for yourself or a loved one or it could mean having a health issue that pushes you out of the job market.

People are hurt and confused and in many cases their only motivation is making sure that their loved ones don't suffer because of what happened. When forced to choose between paying energy bills, paying for medicine, and paying for food, many people cut their food spending first.

They eat less to make ends meet, or stretch their dollars by buying more low-cost, low nutrition—yet highly caloric—"junk" foods.

SNAP benefits help prevent this nutritional risk. What do participants buy with SNAP benefits? Vegetables, fruit, grain products, meat and meat alternatives account for three-quarters of the value of products purchased. As far as value is concerned, 83% of benefits in 2010 were redeemed in supermarkets or super stores. Ninety six percent of SNAP households shop at a supermarket or super store at some time during each month.[43]

You can see the allowable locations by going to http://www.snapretailerlocator.com/. Farmers' Markets are becoming a more common place for benefits to be redeemed. You can see which markets are approved at http://foodconvo.com/SQgN2M.

Sometimes you hear reports about abuse of SNAP benefits, but there is no legal way to convert benefits into cash. The USDA takes abuse attempts very seriously, and trafficking in cash conversion of benefits is below one percent.

Do people in need of food assistance deserve to know where their food comes from? Are they likely to have different hot buttons? Will you learn just as much from them as you would from having a conversation with a Whole Foods customer? Absolutely! Given the amount of time we spend talking about feeding 9 billion people by 2050, those living in food insecurity form a critical segment to understand.

Farms and ranches are in the business of raising products that are or will be turned into food. Agriculture is in the business of supporting that venture. Let's be sure we're talking with all types of influencers, whether they're young or old, well off or on SNAP, in the city or next door—and finding out what's important to them. This does not have to be difficult or time consuming.

Hot buttons bring people to the table

A hot button is something that really grabs a person's attention; it could be a need, an interest, or a passion. Learning others' hot buttons is a step many try to skip, I've found. You will miss a key opportunity if you don't work at identifying hot buttons—even if you know the person well. The value is in understanding others rather than operating from assumptions.

Before you start trying to push buttons, make sure you know who you're talking to and what's important to them—though it may not be obvious. **If you are successful in uncovering hot buttons, you'll find that hand extended across the plate much more quickly.**

I am convinced the answer to sharing the farm story is in our ability to more closely connect the people around the plate. Finding hot buttons is a straightforward approach to turning a daunting task into simply relating to people. Why don't you go to your targeted influencer group today, ask questions, and find their hot buttons?

CHAPTER 3

Why? Translate Farm to Fork by Speaking Their Language

"I've learned that people will forget what you said, people will forget what you did, but people will never forget how you made them feel."
- Maya Angelou

Have you ever tried to speak Chinese to your neighbor or had a worker communicate with you in only Spanish? It's a tough proposition, isn't it? The same is true when people in agriculture try to speak "ag" to the food side of the plate—confusion results.

In order to successfully connect why should agriculture should matter to the person you're trying to connect with, you have to serve as the translator. A common mistake we make in agriculture is to "data dump" soon as we get a chance. We talk about science, research, or what we want to get across as soon as we can.

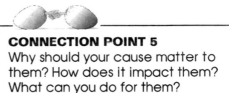

CONNECTION POINT 5
Why should your cause matter to them? How does it impact them? What can you do for them?

When we data dump, we lose the chance to connect. Why? Because it needs to be about them, not you. Invest time early in the conversation to learn about the other person's interests and values. Your goal is to continue growing rapport while getting to know more about the other's hot buttons and translating agriculture slowly to their interests.

In other words, **make them feel good rather than pummeling them with facts!** Don't puke data on their shoes. Here are a few quick tips to get them interested enough to move the conversation to another level:

- Keep the other person actively talking, and be concerned about his or her needs and interests; you'll make that person feel special!

- Actively listen by responding through body language, rephrasing what the other person said to confirm understanding, and asking follow—up questions.
- Identify whether you're dealing with an emotional or rational person and which personality type they fall into.
- Share basic information—just enough to whet the appetite.

What can you discuss that will really push the buttons of your target audience? This may be as simple as giving a child milk and cookies or as complicated as addressing animal welfare issues with a pet owner or discussing the use of technology on farms at the grocery store.

Farming fun in the classroom

Sarah Bedgar Wilson is a former Maryland dairy queen who now farms with her husband, Jeremy, and three young children in North Dakota. They've seen more than their share of challenges getting started farming, but Sarah always makes the time to tell their story. She shared her experiences with translating agriculture through the hot buttons of kids and teachers:

- *Take accurate ag books and read them and leave a few behind for the classroom and school libraries. Ideally, each child can keep one too. I work with the author/publisher to try to get a bulk discount.*
- *Plan on hands-on activities, too—examples of crops and making butter in a jar, etc.*
- *Bring each child an "I met a farmer today" sticker. That way, they talk to their parents about my visit at home.*
- *Consider summers as a great time to work with libraries and daycares. Schools often have summer or after—school programs that would love visitors, as well.*
- *See http://foodconvo.com/PWyW1Q for more ideas.*
- *Work with commodity groups, too, to get soybean crayons or coloring books, honey sticks, etc. donated to match the crop or season you're talking about.*

As far as preschool and early elementary school hot buttons, make it fun. Let them share their experiences with food and farming. I always try to make any farm kids in the group feel really proud and special. They always love the game where I take a bucket of household items and try to guess the crop/animal they came from.

Teacher hot buttons center around how you can make their job easy by matching your visit and lessons to their curriculum and schedule. Give them an exact time of arrival/departure and stick to it. Leave them the same goodie bag the kids got—they love that! Leave teacher with links to future lesson ideas and book lists.

You can see how easily Sarah translates agriculture through hot buttons of these two influencer groups. She's used that same approach to bring other farmers and ranchers into the fold to share agriculture's story, as you'll find at http://farmeronamission.blogspot.com.

Why do you have two ears and one mouth?

We have two ears to listen closely with, yet we often spend more time focusing on what's going to glide off of our golden tongues. Although I do like to talk (what professional speaker doesn't?), I believe we were given 32 teeth to hold our one tongue in place while we put our two ears to use.

In other words, **spend time preparing insightful questions that will help you get to know the other person** instead of worrying about how you're going to data dump about how fabulous agriculture is. Consider how annoying it is to deal with salespeople who dominate the conversation and focus more on their pitches than on the customers—don't make the same mistake in connecting.

> **ROTTEN VEGETABLE 5**
> Are you using foul language? Genetically modified organisms. Factory farms. Industrial agriculture. High fructose corn syrup. The agricultural industry. Agriculture is ripe with terms that scare people. We are responsible for some of those terms, whereas activists coined others. Can you talk about your farm, biotechnology, and the business of agriculture, progress, and different farm practices? Words matter—especially when you're talking to those outside of our business.

Ask thought-provoking questions and <u>listen</u> to the answers if you want to improve your chance of going beyond the choir. Leave a scar in your tongue if you have to, but spend more time using those two ears than anything else!

Let's start with an influencer group you're likely to agree with because they share similar hot buttons. My research shows that dietitians are concerned with credibility for their profession, recommendations coming from those without training, public acceptance of science, and dispelling myths. Sound familiar?

Science is the common language of farm and nutrition

Donna Manring, DTR, provides an inside view of the nutrition professional's world. She is the owner and founder of Innovative Dining Solutions and has many years in the food industry specializing in nutrition, dietetics, leadership, customer service, and operational improvement. Donna believes food is one of life's greatest pleasures, is a proud mom and /grandma, and loves to spend time in the kitchen.

Today it seems agriculture and nutrition is more complicated than when I was a kid. If you look in the dictionary for the definition of nutrition and agriculture, you will see similarities. Included in both is "science and application of those principals." Information technology is shaping agricultural/nutritional science and its application, often stating inadequate and misleading information by those wishing to sell products or advance their own agenda.

The need for reliable sources of scientific data is growing, as consumers are growing tired of misinformation. At the basis of public concern is a feeling of not being fully informed or, worse, of not being told the truth. Nutrition professionals (accredited by Academy of Nutrition and Dietetics) are continually addressing nutrition myths and fallacies. The agriculture industry experiences these same challenges. It

CONNECTION POINT 6

Influencer Groups	Example Hot Buttons
Consumers	Food safety convenience, cost
Media	Expert sources, timeliness, community interest
Schools	State standards, respect, ease of use, funding, lunch nutrition program
Children	Fun, popularity, what's "cool"
Civic organizations	Visibility, serving community needs, membership, quality of life, their "cause"

becomes frustrating when dealing with inaccuracies and broad-based statements that defy science.

Take for example, high fructose corn syrup (HFCS); science clearly proves that HFCS is metabolized similarly as cane sugar, yet there are those that state what is a negative "opinion," and it is not science based information. Every day there will be someone who touts a "belief" or a headline that clearly is not science-based. Whether it is gluten free, dairy free or whatever the headline may be, we in agriculture and nutrition are the resources to clear the confusion.

Nutrition and agriculture have similar, if not the same, hot buttons. Without a doubt, we are passionate about our role in providing science-based information. I get excited when I think about nutrition and agriculture working together as a respected aligned culture of professionals advancing awareness and encouraging consumers to refer to reputable resources for information.

Together, we have shared objectives and many opportunities to collaborate on methods, tools, and mechanisms to work together. Today, more than ever, the commitment is strong to tackle hunger, food safety, and nutrition through agriculture. Let's pledge to continue to build an innovative partnership and strengthen our link in order to deliver opti-

mal nutrition and agriculture information. By seeking closer collaboration with nutrition, agriculture can gain new insights into the needs of its primary customer, the consumer. The question is not whether there should be a closer relationship between agriculture and nutrition, but rather how best to achieve it.

The Academy of Nutrition and Dietetics (AND) is the world's largest organization of food and nutrition professionals. AND is committed to improving the nation's health and advancing the profession of dietetics through research, education, and advocacy. Collaboration between nutrition and agriculture communities will allow the opportunity to share information, resulting in a strategic alliance. Social networking keeps me informed and enhances my knowledge base with the agriculture community. Attending the World Dairy Expo was a huge eye—opener for me. It was informative, and it was an incredible learning experience. How will you learn more about nutrition and agriculture?

As a nutrition professional, I will be looking to connect with agriculture to better understand ways to work together. Will you join me?

I sure hope you'll take Donna and others up on their interest in connecting with farmers, ranchers, and the other people of agriculture. The more I go beyond the choir, the more I'm amazed at how interested people are in connecting with the humans in our business.

The beauty of the 6 ½ steps to the farm side of the conversation is that it can be done in person or online. "Agvocacy" is a term used to describe agricultural advocacy—telling your story-in social media spaces (this is covered more in Chapters 5 and 6).

Connecting as a human, not a farmer

A farmer in Nebraska, Zach Hunnicutt, shares how he translates farming to connect with hot buttons through Twitter, Facebook, and Instagram. Interestingly enough, he doesn't talk a lot about farming as he's developing relationships—it's more about human interest stories like football and Oscar dresses.

CONNECTION POINT 2
You're less likely to experience rejection if you're appealing to people's hot buttons. This is about them, not you. If you stay focused on their interests, you'll forget your own fear.

When the University of Nebraska moved to the Big Ten, I did all I could to drill this information into your eyeballs while the whole conference-realignment business was at its fever pitch. Because of the magical convergence of GPS auto steer in my tractor, a smartphone, and long days applying fertilizer, I could follow and share all the information the internet had to offer about which school was going where and which conferences might collapse. To say I was obsessed would be understating the fact; to say I was annoying wouldn't be incorrect.

What does this have to do with telling the farming story? Everything. Not because Nebraska is a land-grant university whose agricultural research will be greatly aided by entry into the Big Ten, and not because some cutting-edge ag technology made it happen, but because it allowed my followers to see a human element to the farmer behind the smartphone.

One of the chief aims of agvocates is to reconnect a disconnected public with their food production. At a basic level, this means making sure that people know that milk and eggs aren't made at the grocery store, that field corn and sweet corn are different, and that somebody has to butcher the meat they're grilling, to name a few issues (I can't count the number of times I've explained that popcorn isn't just yellow corn that pops). It also means explaining what we do and why, to clear up misconceptions and give the public a greater understanding of what we're doing on the farm.

However, we need to remember that we're not just connecting The Public with The Farm. Social media is about connecting Zach in Nebraska with Jesse in New Jersey. Agvocacy becomes most effective when we add that human voice to the farm. For instance, I obsess over sports like a lot of my followers. I deal with the same joys and frustrations of parenting. Somehow, I even got sucked into watching the Oscars (and tweeting about a dress, no less...).

Basically, I'm a human being like anyone else, I just work on the production end of the food supply. And once people know Zach the person along with Zach the farmer, I (hopefully) earn a higher level of trust when I talk about agriculture. Just as we trust offline friends to recommend things such as music and restaurants, developing online relationships builds a trust that can make all the difference in sharing your agvocacy story.

So there's my deeply insightful advice for agvocates out there: talk about your lives. Tweet about your favorite music. Obsess over your sports teams on Facebook. Share what you're seeing while people-watching in malls and airports (just remember it's a public forum...and hope that lady with the mullet isn't on Twitter). Take a picture and post it on Instagram. Focus on making a human connection with your audience while you're conversing—and you may be given the opportunity to make an educational connection.

Zach provides a good perspective on some fun ways to humanize the farming story by connecting to other people with hot buttons such as sports, parenting, and fashion. Just for the record, Zach is part of a large, progressive corn and soybean operation in Nebraska and worked at a commodity brokerage before returning to the family farm.

He's a proud dad of two small kiddos, and his wife, Anna, is also active in growing connections for agriculture. Their family graces the cover of Chapter 2 on the food side of this book. They serve on the American Farm Bureau Young Farmers & Ranchers committee and are smart enough to realize that human connections will ultimately determine the success of their business—and likely that of their children.

Zach also brings perspective to the power of social media sites such as Facebook, Twitter, YouTube, Linkedin, Pinterest, Instagram, and many more that I won't mention because they'll change before this book is printed.

Translating ag talk may seem as difficult as learning another language. It's not. It simply requires practice and will feel a bit awkward at first, but it sure beats vomiting science, research, and technical jargon on the 98.5% of society that's not on a farm.

Can you speak the language of the influencers you're focusing on? Are you doing so in advance of crises, or are you simply reacting?

CHAPTER 4

When? Fifteen Minutes Daily Building Engagement

"Reactive people focus on circumstances over which they have no control. The negative energy generated by that focus, combined with neglect in areas they could do something about, causes their circle of influence to shrink. Proactive people focus their efforts on the things they can do something about. The nature of their energy is positive, enlarging, and magnifying, causing their circle of influence to increase."
~ Stephen Covey

Positive energy that increases your circle of influence sounds great, right? Then take the time to connect with people around the food plate before the next crisis! Why wait for the next animal rights video, media misinformation, or food claim such as that about pink slime? What if you took personal responsibility for investing 15 minutes each day to proactively connect with people?

Are you fouling out or scoring points?

Is the game of basketball won on points or defense? No surprise to anyone who knows me, but my basketball-playing days usually included some hardcore defense and fouling out, thanks to a few well-placed hip bumps and elbows. One of the many things I love about Michigan State University's basketball strategy is tough defense. Coach Tom Izzo, worthy of an entire book on leadership, is known for getting more excited about missed rebounds than missed shots.

The only way the game is won is to get some points on the board, however. No points means no win, which translates the priority to offense—and if you've ever played basketball, you know good offense takes a lot of practice. It's no different for agriculture.

We've had a lot of practice playing defense, running down the court chasing the latest claims about animal abuse and environmental disaster. I've seen thousands of agricultural folks quickly rise up and defend our practices against activist claims, pulling out every fact, piece of research, and study. Then they wonder why they "foul out" as the information falls on deaf ears. I suggest you analyze the "game clips" of activists to find that answer—**emotion trumps science in nearly every play.**

With no crisis to defend, however, thousands in agriculture sit back without a care about offense. If the only way the game is won is to get points on the board, it's pretty clear that automatically sets agriculture up for a loss. Why is it so difficult to talk to your neighbors about what drives you to farm the way you do, to share photos on Facebook, to talk to the media, or to develop relationships with elected officials when there is no crisis? **Is it impossible for us to be proactive and look beyond playing defense?**

Offense matters. My research over the past decade clearly shows that when a person can name a farmer and refer to that farm's practices, it mitigates the person's reaction to activist claims. In other words, when the next nasty animal rights video comes out, if Suzy Q consumer can say, "I know Francine Farmer up the road and believe in what she does. She doesn't treat her animals or land like that. I don't think this video is right," That's a win for agriculture—and no energy needs to be wasted on defense. Equally as important, the focus stays positive, allowing the discussion to happen with decorum.

Just to be clear, the typical conversation around food and farming should <u>not</u> be a win/lose scenario. **Our goal should be handshakes across the food plate and understanding that we'll have to agree to disagree at times.**

Will the media tell your story?

Are you waiting for the media to tell your story? Hoping that you might suddenly see major networks espousing farmers? Thinking a paid spokesperson will do it for you or that ag media professionals will do it for you?

None of those are going to happen, so how about you reach out a hand out to those outside of agriculture? Pick your targeted influencer group and begin a proactive conversation. As the next contributor points out, no one—including media—can do that more effectively than you.

Susan Crowell is the editor of *Farm and Dairy* newspaper (www.farmanddairy. com) in Salem, Ohio. A mom to two college students, Susan has been known to rant about poor spelling and grammar. She enjoys writing stories to help farmers, but not to tell their stories. You see, she doesn't believe you need her to tell your story.

I'm a farm journalist. A writer. Telling stories is what I do best. No, not tall tales, but the stories of everyday people, the stories of how laws and policies affect farm folks, and the stories of great joy and unbelievable heartache—the stories of life.

Stories are powerful, because people pay attention to stories. Facts are boring, statistics are boring, lectures are boring, sermons are boring. But stories? We sit up and listen. Storytelling pulls in people with real-world pictures and sounds and scents. Stories create connections.

Your participation in social media—by commenting on online blogs or articles, by starting conversations with strangers on Twitter, or by sharing your farm story on a blog— is powerful because your voice, the voice of "real" farmers, manure-splashed-boots-on-the-ground farmers, is the voice everyone wants to hear. They don't want to listen to me, I'm just the middleman. They want to listen to you.

When you want a recommendation for a nice restaurant, who do you turn to? Most likely, your friends or family. But in today's age, you might also turn to your social media networks, because you've come to "know" these people, even those you've never met face-to-face.

You have that same value and trust to individuals in your social networks, in return. Your stories can make agriculture come alive to a single parent in metropolitan Chicago. Your stories can bridge gaps between farm and non—farm residents, between organic and conventional producers and supporters.

Your voice, your stories, give these other groups a bigger lens through which they can now view agriculture. Just like sharing a story at the coffee shop with the city councilman. Only, your "local community" is as wide and deep as you want to make it. As you make those connections, a wonderful thing happens: conversations. Questions. And answers. Jokes. Suggestions. And, yes, challenges and prodding.

You are a living, breathing farmer, and your passion can impact others more than the cold, hard facts. You know, the boring stuff. There's a reason the USDA developed its "Know Your Farmer, Know Your Food"[44] campaign. It's called "putting a face on agriculture."

Social media brings us life on speed. We are connected to each other in nanoseconds. Things that used to take years now happen in minutes. News travels quicker than heifers find open gates. We have larger platforms to get points across, more quickly than ever before.

As Associated Press writer Andrew Welsh-Huggins tweeted: "1st day thought from Kiplinger social media program: moving from 'Mass Communication to Massive Communication.'"

Agriculture needs to be in that arena of "massive communication." Conversations are taking place, with or without you—conversations that impact public opinion and public policy.

We're in a new media world order. Consumers don't need me (a traditional journalist) anymore (well, yes, they do, but that's for another day!), when they can get their stories from you.

The great thing about social media is that it's not just a one-way street. Through it, farmers can look for other voices to learn from and grow with: mommy bloggers, gardeners, foodies, and yes, even journalists. They have stories to tell, too.

Don't think this new media world order is out of your league, because it's not. You don't have to learn it all, but you do have to dip your toe in the water to get started.

Helen Keller said: "I am only one, but still I am one. I cannot do everything, but still I can do something; and because I cannot do everything, I will not refuse to do the something that I can do."

The world is waiting to hear your side of the story.

Media, rejection, and other farmer fears

I realize you may dread talking to the media—even if it's people in the ag media like Susan. In working with agricultural audiences across North America, I find that around 90% want nothing to do with mainstream media, yet the reality is that people all around the food plate are using the media to talk about farming, food, ranches, and farmers. **Should you really complain about the conversation if you're not willing to take part?**

Most people will respond that the media will make them look stupid, misquote them, or make their farm a target. I always ask if they think they're guaranteed none of those things are going to happen if they refuse to serve as expert sources. I actually think it boils down to the fear of rejection. No is one of the most feared words in the English language—these two little letters can strike fear in even the strongest of people.

ROTTEN VEGETABLE 6
Letting others do the talking for farmers and ranchers. According to the book How Risky Is It, Really?, people are more afraid of business & industry, politicians, and processes that are closed and. are less afraid (more likely to trust) consumer groups, neutral experts, and processes that are open.

If you get a cold no, it's a likely indicator that you probably didn't spend enough time learning about the other person's needs, so transfer some of your energy from complaining to learning. Then get over the personal rejection factor. "No" probably didn't cause you physical pain from having the door slammed in your face (if that happened, I suggest a communications class).

"No" simply means that you didn't hit the other person's hot buttons (see Chapter 3) and need to go back asking questions. Here are some ways to graciously deal with objections:

CONNECTION POINT 8
You don't have to be loud or obnoxious or even know good jokes to be the life of the party in connecting agriculture! True interest in the person you're talking to, good listening skills, and keen observation will quickly make you interesting enough to be remembered.

- Let the person know you'd like to better understand.
- Restate the objection to be sure you heard it correctly.
- Ask questions that drill down to the real issue. The stated objection may not be the real issue!
- Provide facts or personal experience to back up your claims if necessary.
- Bring laughter to the conversation.

Face it—objections are a part of doing business today. Just remember to keep your cool and continue asking questions—go back to step two and identify hot buttons! I've been told no in several different languages and am proof that "no" won't kill you! Look at no as standing for "new opportunity"—your chance to step back and do some more exploring.

Also remember that objections can be more subtle than the word no. They can be found in the rejection of a choice, the tone of voice, or the manner in which the conversation is approached. **The worst rejection I've witnessed is turning food into the new politics and religion — topics not to be discussed in public. We all lose if food becomes that contentious.**

Playing on food emotions

Jennifer Elwell in Kentucky offers great perspective both on telling your story and dealing with objections. She's worked as a communications professional in agriculture for quite some time but began blogging on her own a few years ago. The movie *Food, Inc.* lit her fire to speak out in support of modern agriculture.

> **ROTTEN VEGETABLE 7**
> Waiting too long to explain the reality of farming today. Why do many city dwellers have the a romanticized view of how their food is produced and a negative image of "mega- farms"? Perhaps because we haven't told them differently.

Through blogging and the social media space, Jennifer has learned how to handle objections and different ways of thinking. As a result, Jennifer has been invited to participate in food and mommy blogger conferences to share the farm perspective, clearly showing her ability to rise above screeching on an airplane. More importantly, it's given her the chance to learn from the food and mommy blogger community.

Like it or not, food is an emotional subject for many people. It can bring happiness and fond memories but can also quite easily cause fear. Good or bad, a lot of people wanting to share information about food like to play on these emotions. Whether or not a person will internalize or act on the information they receive depends a lot on their individual experiences. Realizing that we don't all think about food the same way was my breakthrough moment, and it significantly altered my approach to having food conversations.

I have worked in agricultural business for 15 years. For the longest time, I knew all the "right" things to say and found myself getting extremely frustrated when someone had an alternate opinion. One of my earliest memories of a food conversation happened on an airplane. I sat next to a woman who said she only purchased organic eggs. Unfortunately, I remember responding with some form of "that's stupid" and people began to stare because my voice continued to get louder and louder.

Fast-forward to a conversation 14 years later, I am again sitting on an airplane. I discover that the woman beside me shares my love for fashion and shoes, and I eventually find a way to drop in that I love my job working for farmers (yes, I definitely have a passion for what I do). She was then quick to tell me that she was a vegan. I didn't get mad, and I didn't jump to the conclusion that she had a mental disorder for not embracing my meat-eating culture.

We continued to have meaningful conversation. I learned that she grew up on a grain and beef cattle farm but adopted her behaviors at a very young age because of her love for animals. I learned that she had friends who had serious health problems that doctors related to eating too much meat.

I also learned that many vegans are careful to label their eating habits because other vegans are watching very closely and will be quick to call them on their mistakes. In the end, she still told me she loved my leather shoes. I figured out that this was not the time to question someone's eating habits. She had very personal reasons for making those choices. She was not quoting me facts she had heard, just sharing her experiences.

Today, I critically think about why there are so many differing opinions about food. I never make assumptions, and I ask questions instead of talking at people. I also rarely lead my questions with "why" because it puts many people on the defensive if they think I am questioning their judgment.

Once the conversation starts to move along, I begin to share my experiences and make it clear that I feel a certain way because of my experiences. This opens so many doors for people to ask me questions, and many of those questions start with "why," which I am glad to answer.

In the end, there may still be people who want to be vegans, or only buy organic, or continue to make daily trips to their favorite fast-food restaurant. Our food system can meet all of these desires.

I no longer believe it is my mission to change behaviors, but to just share some of my knowledge of agriculture and what farmers are doing. My daily goal is to erase fear one may have about food and hope that decisions will be made with a bit of understanding.

Jennifer shares her journey in figuring out what is the best way to feed her family, the joys and struggles of trying to produce food herself, her appreciation for the famers who provide food, and her beliefs on what is real and what is hype regarding our food supply http://foodmommy.blogspot.com. She's not only helping give a voice to farmers but also sharing a guilt-free approach with other moms. That's reaching across the food plate!

When should you be making an effort to reach across the food plate? Any time in the day, for 15 minutes per day. It does not have to be as complicated as writing a blog—it can be taking time to talk about what you do and why your farm the way you do in the church parking lot. It can be putting up pictures of your combine or newborn baby calf with a couple of quick explanations on Facebook. It could be going into a classroom, tweeting from the toilet, making a legislative visit, —or— gasp—talking to the media!

As Covey said, "Proactive people focus their efforts on the things they can do something about. The nature of their energy is positive, enlarging, and magnifying, causing their circle of influence to increase." What can you do something about?

Please realize that agriculture is losing in the courtroom of public opinion if you choose not to be proactive. **Reach across the plate for 15 minutes per day.** I dare you to try it for a month and see what happens! 🌾

CHAPTER 5

Where? Think Global, Act Local

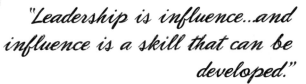

"Leadership is influence...and influence is a skill that can be developed."

~ John Maxwell

Big picture. It's easy to lose sight of when you're worried about the minutiae of managing your animals, planning for the next planting, and running a business, yet we have to make the time to look at the big picture view of agriculture.

Research shows that food buyers assume food will be safe, healthy, and affordable—and they believe those should be priorities for all farms, large and small. They want also want you to prioritize humane treatment of farm animals and make the environment cleaner, healthier, and safer.[45]

Call me crazy, but **today's regulations and activist agendas will impact you—your family, your bottom line, your right to farm**—in five or ten years, if not sooner. Are you sure that you don't have time to step up and connect with others around the food plate? Of course you need to take care of home fires, but don't do so at the demise of the big picture of agriculture.

CONNECTION POINT 9
Scripted folks come off as less than genuine. Farmers sharing their authentic stories, even of large family operations, are considered authentic. Transparency about what you really do on your farm or ranch trumps any argument. Transparency can be incredibly hard to define, but it involves an honest discussion about what's right and wrong in today's agriculture.

Farm and food connections happen at any time, any place

Let's not make this more complicated than it needs to be: you can have a conversation to connect food and farming anywhere, in just a few minutes. For example, one Sunday after church, we went with family friends to have ice cream at a favorite hangout. As we watched our daughters on the playground, concerns over girls developing too early came up.

"What's the deal with hormones and antibiotics in milk? Are all of the concerns legitimate?" our friends asked. My ruminant nutritionist husband and I explained that all food has hormones in it and always has. We also talked through how milk is tested at the farm, when it arrives at the plant, and when it's bottled and gave them a quick overview of the USDA's Grade A standards.

> **ROTTEN VEGETABLE 8**
> Do we sometimes get so hung up on bringing recognition to farmers that we lose sight of bringing recognition to millions of others who share responsibility for food, fuel, feed, and fiber? I'll be the first one to say that the non-farm public needs to talk to a farmer or rancher if they want to learn about food, but the reality is that many are responsible—and are just as important to food production—as food producers. With all due respect to farmers and ranchers, there is a need for all parts of the food system to be understood. That includes agribusinesses, meat scientists, food technicians, and many others.

"That makes sense." was the response from our friends, who happen to be bank and medical executives. They measured this information with their own education and their personal experience with a daughter who drinks a whole lot of milk without any health issues—and they were perfectly comfortable. **A meaningful conversation really can be that simple.**

Another example comes from Ryan, a passionate agricultural advocate from down south. He's originally from Arkansas and is currently pursuing his master's degree at the University of Tennessee. Ryan loves a good steak and is glad to talk about it to anyone he comes across, yet he targets his conversations and approaches them through common values, even when CNN invited him to blog on Eatocracy.

Opportunities for conversations about food and farming exist everywhere I turn, but that was not something I recognized from the start. Seeking out these conversation starters takes some practice and a little effort at first, but over time, it becomes easier to join a discussion.

As a college student, I find the university campus full of opportunities for food dialogues. Although most college students are quite confident in their opinions, campus is a learning environment that makes listening to others easier to do. I have conversations about food and farming with my circle of friends and classmates on a regular basis, but the most encouraging engagements come with those outside of my comfort zone.

One example of these conversations is the Food Policy group at the University of Tennessee. This is a group of students with ideas about food that greatly differ from my own.

However, we are able to have great discussions about food options with questions stemming from both sides of the table.

I find starting conversations with others is made easier when we have mutual interests outside of those topics on the table for discussion. Being able to start the conversations with topics where we may have more common ground or previous relationships makes the tougher, more heated topics easier to approach. Some of the most productive food and farming conversations and questions come from those who surround me on a regular basis—family, friends, coworkers, church members, neighbors.

When the opportunity is not available to establish relationships or mutual interests prior to food or farming conversations, I find it best to do more listening and asking of questions before sharing my opinion. We can learn a lot about someone just by asking about their opinions. Save the more in-depth questions for later on during the conversation.

In the world of food and farming conversations, many people will comment for the sake of having something to say. When a question or comment comes with some form of accusation, I take a moment for background reading to understand better the position of the commenter.

If online, utilize back-links, previous conversations, or profile information to learn more about where the person is coming from. If in person, look for nonverbal cues to recognize sarcasm or genuine interest. This will help a lot in learning how to approach the conversation. Most of the time, if the comment or question comes from someone with lack of interest in actual conversation, I may respond to be polite and only continue correspondence if replies are cordial.

My best advice when approaching conversations about food or farming, whether online or in person boils down to 5 points.

- *Be real and authentic about your passion for agriculture.*
- *Show enthusiasm for your passion.*
- *Keep it simple and to the point.*
- *Make it a candid point of view.*
- *Stick to your experience; you can't defend everyone.*

You can learn more from Ryan's experiences reaching out to tell agriculture's story at http://agricultureproud.com.

Innocent questions or skepticism about farming?

Another approach is to bring people to your farm for a tour, picnic, or open house. Nieman Farms in Iowa has feeder cattle, a cow/calf herd, wean-to-finish hogs, corn, soybeans, and hay and shares its agricultural advocacy experience after hosting a community open house. It's a great perspective about how defensive farmers can be when people start asking questions.

Last fall our family held an open house to celebrate our newly constructed confinement hoop barn for our feeder cattle. We went out of our way to invite non-farm neighbors, members of our church, acquaintances, and the broader community in general. We learned that some questions are just that—and it's important to not respond defensively.

"So, the cattle don't ever go outside?" was a question I received from one of the attendees. She had no farm experience. Now, I am all too familiar with the nasty accusations that can be hurled at certain farming practices. There are individuals who feel it is cruel to keep an animal under a roof while it is being fattened for market—and they are none too hesitant to share their feelings. I've been round and round with people, and despite my best efforts, some minds just can't be changed.

I'll admit, my defenses immediately went up at the asking of this question. I assumed that she disapproved of the practice. For a second, I considered a snarky response. Then I took a step back. She was simply asking an innocent question, and if I responded with a short answer, I would have the absolute wrong effect.

I explained that, yes, the cattle get to spend the rest of their lives being pampered in this barn, with fresh bedding added weekly and daily balanced meals delivered right to their feed bunk. They would be monitored closely for health and comfort, as a happy calf is a productive calf. I told her if she wanted to learn more, she could follow our farm on my blog.

In face-to-face conversations and online comment threads, I have occasionally seen a different scenario play out. A farmer will become defensive in explanations of the practices they use on their farm and will resort to an accusatory tone, especially if the individual they are talking with disapproves. The conversation spirals downward from there, and neither party is working to find common ground. While I understand this reaction to criticism, I also realize that becoming defensive is counterproductive when sharing the great message of agriculture.

My philosophy as an "agvocate" is to remember that most of the people I talk to, even the ones who disagree with me, are simply looking for information. It's my job to provide that information while finding common ground. I don't have to agree with someone in order to respect them. I let my commitment to my work show, check my attitude frequently, and build a bridge.

When engaging in discussions about agriculture in food production, remember to ask yourself, innocent question or skepticism? When in doubt, treat it as an innocent question, show the other person that you are a respectable human being, and maybe, just maybe, you'll begin to build that bridge.

We have a tendency to think people are stupid, putting their noses where they don't belong, or are against modern agriculture, when, in fact, neither is true. **Where are you likely to get the most defensive?**

How can you set up roadblocks for yourself to remember that many times, people are simply seeking more information about their food? Remember, if you don't provide information where they'd like it, in a way that's digestible for them, they'll seek answers elsewhere.

Throughout this book, you've seen references to tools in our highly social world, such as Twitter, Facebook, YouTube, Klout, blogging, Pinterest, and Linkedin. I know some readers wish the whole social media thing would just disappear. I could tell you that Facebook reached 150 million users nearly five times faster than cell phones did or point to my research that shows anti-agriculture activist groups growing their social media presence 150-fold in four years, but I'll let another farmer, Ryan Weeks, explain why social media is a huge opportunity for agriculture.

Ryan is a middle-aged farmer in northern Nebraska, plays big in the seed business as a dealer, and is the proud dad to three kids, who frequent his combine cab. He also posts pictures of his iPad in the tractor cab and loves anything to do with technology—and Husker football. He and his wife, Kristi, raise yellow corn, popcorn, soybeans, alfalfa, and prairie hay on the family farm settled by his family in the late 1800s.

Their operation prides itself on quick adaptation of technology, being stewards of the land they farm, and helping in the community in which they live. Ryan wrote the following post a few years ago, but it still speaks to why farmers need to engage in these "newfangled" tools.

Yes, you really do need to Facebook, tweet or blog

Why did I get involved with social media? Was it a dream of mine to get banned from the HSUS Twitter account since I was a little kid? Nope. I found the misinformation being spread about farming and ranching on sites such as YouTube as a problem that needed to have a counter argument.

Of course, I first signed on to Facebook to connect with friends, but it quickly moved to agvocacy when I saw non-factual information being taken as fact regarding farming practices. Specifically, agriculture was being blamed for a lot of problems (diabetes, obesity, etc) in our society that I felt are about consumption, not production.

I knew for quite awhile what would result from "factory farming" searches on YouTube and had seen the smokestacks in the background of a cornfield in the movie Food, Inc. This really hit me —I have a passion for what we do in agriculture and have been to third world countries where food choice is not an option. You eat what you have, if you have anything.

Labeling our food production system as broken when we are feeding our own, exporting and raising more product on fewer inputs made me want to start speaking up. I have always spoken locally about economic impacts of agriculture, specifically animal ag, but the national conversation has nothing to do with economics. It has everything to do with emotion. Science, no matter how factual, has a hard time trumping emotion. Heartfelt messages always win.

I felt there needed to be a farmer voice in social media conversations about agriculture. My social media journey started with Facebook, graduated to Twitter, then I created a Facebook page for our farm, and then started using Linkedin and YouTube. It seems like quite a lot, but with apps like TweetDeck, it becomes manageable. It has afforded me the opportunity to go the AgChat Foundation conference (a phenomenal grassroots organization) and be around a tremendous group of family farmers to improve our skills in social media.

The best thing that's happened in this journey is a chance to converse with more consumers about the advantages and disadvantages of certain aspects of our food system in an environment that usually contains mutual respect. There are antagonists and misunderstandings, but the beauty of most social media products is that you have the ability to hit block, ignore, or have a community of agvocates support you. We all are working together to support each other—something that doesn't always happen in agriculture.

Most recently we entered the world of blogging at www.cornhuskerfarmer.word press.com and I have found that to write, you need inspiration. This usually means that I have to be driven by emotion. I have tried to start jotting down ideas on my phone when they come to me and then approaching them later, but the most effective seems to be writing in the heat of the moment.

I hope many more in agriculture will start having the conversations about our farms and ranches in any of these mediums. We need all of you!

If you think for one minute you can't make a difference or that your voice isn't needed, search "factory farming" on YouTube and see what comes up—and then tell me we don't need you. Whose voice is countering the misinformation? If not you, then who?

Why did I get involved? Because no one else is going to tell my story! Who is telling your farm story? Take the time to learn these new tools the same way you've adapted to technology in your equipment.

Nothing beats face-to-face communications, but you won't be able reach one billion people at your local coffee shop or at the end of your driveway. As of the writing of this book, that's how many people are on Facebook. Pinterest is changing online shopping. News is being broken and sourced on Twitter every second of the day. **Social media isn't a fad, it's a culture changer.**

The Twitterverse is not outer space

Wayne Black, a cash crop farmer in Ontario, Canada, can tell you more about the tool with a crazy name—Twitter—as he does at http://foodconvo.com/Uyui78.

The biggest reason to be on Twitter or any type of social media is for advocating. It has generated a lot of discussion with politicos, foodies, urbanites and also fellow farmers. My personal use has generated media articles that promote the positive aspects of agriculture and farming in Rural Ontario. People who read my tweets can place a name to a person, which adds value to the message.

The joy of Twitter is that it gives the opportunity to get engaged in a conversation if an issue comes up. You have the opportunity to learn why they have created the negative or positive thought about agriculture. You can walk through a process with the person on the other side to get them engaged in conversation, rather than preaching or appearing to sell the idea.

A lot of times people just want to hear from a farmer. They want to hear what my farm practices are. Understanding why I do what I do gives them further depth to knowing and the ability to question the negative aspects.

Social media allows me as a farmer to become engaged with non-farmers and politicos. We need to become engaged in conversation to get our story out, make it believable and to be truthful. Twitter allows me to do that from wherever I am, in the field, in the barn, in the Boardroom or in my home. People are engaged on the go, even in Rural Ontario.

You may think social media is not for you, but I encourage you to look around. Most likely you'll find a conversation going on that you'll want to weigh in on. Pick a platform and speak up. Let your voice be heard.

Wayne is a great guy and you can catch him at @waynekblack on Twitter. He's involved with several ag and economic development organizations at the local and provincial levels. Wayne also farms with his dad on his family's original farm that dates back to 1867 and enjoys his "wonderful wife and three amazing children."

Don't let these new tools intimidate you. Just as it took you time to adapt to GPS and learn the trials of how it worked best in your fields, it will take time to learn how to best use social media, and it is a tool you learn to use through practice. Twitter has a lingo all its own, but put the crazy terms aside. Try a search for #AgChat, #Farm, #AgNerd or #FoodChat on Twitter to test drive it as a robust search engine (you don't need an account to search). More social media tips and tricks can be found at http://foodconvo.com/RWhHgI.

What about your family and friends?

Over in Chapter 1 on the food side of the book, Jeff VanderWerff shared his experience with people's reactions if he starts a conversation as an apple grower or corn farmer. Jeff's family went back to a more diversified operation when he and his brother wanted to return to the home farm in Michigan, so he straddles the fence between specialty and commodity agriculture.

He provides perspective on the importance of sometimes reaching the hand across the table to our extended family and friends:

Going forward, I would love to find more ways to show the food side of the plate what we are really up to and why we are doing it. I was nearly speechless a few months back, when a good friend of mine from Detroit asked me why we raised corn, when we lose money on it. I was shocked and asked what he meant.

CONNECTION POINT 10
Hone your human skills Everybody has personal interests you can tap into. Some questions help you build rapport no matter where you are:

- What local boards or projects are you involved with?

- Tell me a little bit about your family (relating yours to them will get them to open up).

- I've researched "xyz" about your organization (establishing credibility) and noticed your focus on "xyz" in the future. Can you tell me more about that?

- You have a lot of sports memorabilia. Do you coach or play on a team?

"Well, according to a lot of stuff on the internet, farmers loose money on corn. The government pays you to raise it to prop up ethanol" was his response. I was floored.

Not only was this insulting to me as a businessman, but here was a guy I'd known for close to 15 years, and lived with in college, and I received the impression that he really didn't think we as farmers were astute enough to make our own choices or leave a losing situation.

If this is what people who know me think, what do people who have never even met a farmer believe? It was shocking, almost beyond words to me, even though I've been actively agvocating online and in my community for years. I'm not sure what the answer is, short of posting my profit and loss statements online. However, I am convinced we need to find a way to show folks that we know what we are doing, that we control our own destiny—and that we care about them and what we do.

Jeff offers a solid reminder that we sometimes need to be in conversation with those closest to us. Test his theory out; start a conversation about farming and food at the next holiday gathering you're at—and then let me know what you learn.

Jeff's story is also an illustration that larger farmers need to spend a significant amount of time and energy talking about their values, as **people are skeptical that farmers share their values**. It's also a wake-up call that hot buttons become even more critical as you get larger. Center for Food Integrity research shows that food buyers believe commercial farms' priorities of profitability and productivity are inconsistent with consumer values—food buyers are suspicious of farms that put profit ahead of principle.[46]

Where can you create conversations to translate agriculture? Anywhere! As these examples show, you can make it happen in a coffee shop, in church parking lots, on Facebook, in classrooms, in family conversations, at the PTO, on Capitol Hill, on Twitter, or in civic groups. Figure out where it makes the most sense to reach the influencers you want to engage in the conversation, and meet them there.

Are you influencing the conversation about food? If so, you're helping to lead it, regardless of whether you're conversing in person or online. **Those who lead help determine the course of the conversation.**

CHAPTER 6

How? Follow Your Action Plan

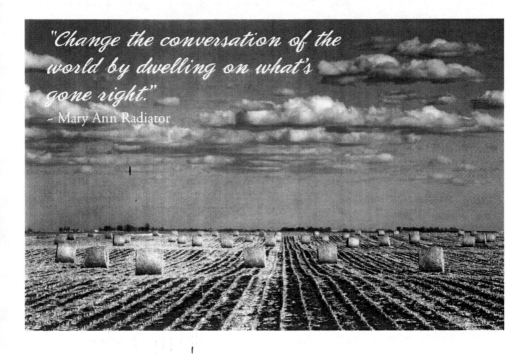

"Change the conversation of the world by dwelling on what's gone right."
~ Mary Ann Radiator

Hopefully, the first five steps raised questions and provided fodder for how to grow your connections around the food plate. Those connections include the people right beside you, those in the same business you're in. Given the independent nature of agriculturists, I don't foresee a day when we all agree.

> **CONNECTION POINT 11**
> Food is an intensely personal choice. It's not our job to tell people that their choices are wrong. It's our job to speak from our side of the food plate and reach across to understand other sides. How are you going to do that?

However, I do expect that we accept—and even embrace—our differences. "United we stand, divided we fall" is a cliché that is all too true with agriculture. Large versus small. Animal versus grain. Organic versus conventional. Pigs versus cows. Corn versus wheat. Look at gestation stalls, rBST, and food versus fuel if you want case studies of the results of agriculture being divided by pundits.

Organic versus conventional is one of the easiest places for farmers to take potshots at each other. I'd like to introduce you to Emily Zweber of Zweber Farms in Minnesota. Emily is a mom to three, loves to bake, and has really amped up their farms' marketing through social media at .http://zweberfarms.com She is also the executive director of the AgChat Foundation, a not-for-profit organization empowering farmers to create connected communities of agvocates. Be sure to check out the foundation's website at http://agchat.org for tips and training on social tools and to join in one of their fast-paced conversations on Twitter, Tuesdays 8-10 p.m. Eastern.

Can farmers work together?

Emily and her husband, Tim, are from "the other side." She shares their experiences with other farmers and their efforts to shake the hands of those beside her, not just of people across the food plate.

ROTTEN VEGETABLE 9
Are your blinders causing you to lose sight of the big picture? Today's regulations and activist agendas will affect you—your family, your bottom line, your right to farm—in five or ten years. Today is the day for you to begin looking at the big picture challenges facing all of agriculture.

When our farm started integrating social media into our risk management strategy in 2009, I was ready as anyone to combat negative comments, misinformation and attacks by those who didn't understand modern agriculture.

Prior to returning to the farm full-time I worked for our state's largest agriculture advocacy organization. I knew all the anti-animal agriculture key messages, their strategy and the like. What I wasn't prepared for was that fellow farmers would be my biggest critics.

Like clockwork each week, a fellow dairy farmer tweets out very nasty and negative things about me and the dairy cooperative we are members of. I have been a called a liar, a hypocrite and been accused of making other dairy farmers suffer because of the way our family farms.

Nothing prepares you emotionally to be criticized by those you consider peers; especially when those peers also choose to attack your family with hurtful and hateful words. I don't wish that on anyone.

You see, on our farm we choose to farm organically. Organic farming works for us. It works for our family, our land and our animals. I am thankful to live in a country where we have such freedoms of choice. I completely understand if this choice in farming method doesn't work for you.

Just as my social media strategy has grown from pure messaging to reaching across the table and creating relationship with customers, so too has my approach with fellow online farmers. Choosing to develop relationships beyond just my commodity and choice in farming method has been very advantageous. I have found many great friends online, both conventional and organic farmers. I have learned a lot by just being open to other points of view. Learning is a two—way street. Oftentimes when I am teaching someone, they are teaching me just as much.

I have made a conscious decision to not close the door on a relationship just because we disagree. It doesn't matter to me if you have 2,000 cows, work for Monsanto, operate a small urban CSA, or just garden with your family. What matters is if you are a person of integrity.

Do you always try to do what is right? Do you care for your family, your animals and your land? That is what matters. Farmers are people. Just like all our customers are people. We might disagree on the issues, but we are still human beings.

So how do farmers of different backgrounds work together? We listen. We respect our individual choices. It is really that simple. None of us have all the answers, but we are each trying to do our best the best way we know how. If you continue to open the doors on relationships, I guarantee that you will learn more than you ever dreamt possible.

Interestingly enough, Emily and I have conversations regularly without any fights. We can civilly talk about the differences in production choices and agree to disagree. My family chooses not to buy organic, but I will advocate for organic farmers like Tim and Emily as much as I would for someone using biotechnology on 5,000 acres. <u>It's about choice in farming.</u> **Consumers are demanding a choice, so why do we find it necessary to begrudge those who choose to farm to meet that demand?**

Challenge yourself beyond the choir

Influencer groups can be reached online and in person. One of my favorite connection examples comes out of Iowa Farm Bureau's leadership program, where I've had the fortune to train agricultural advocates for a decade. We ask each class member to interview three people outside of agriculture and to look up messages from anti-ag activists for in advance of my workshop.

The farmers are typically annoyed or confused by the messaging and misunderstanding around farming they found in their homework. As we walk through the six steps to connecting farm and food, there are predictable outcomes. I'll role play different influencers and see a lot of squirming as the class members are challenged to get out of their comfort zone. There is usually at least one "data dumper" who just can't helping spewing ag information even if no one is listening.

At the end, when I give the groups a little challenge around building bridges with food, the individual groups never work together. Rather, they try to do their own thing. Sound familiar? It's a pretty clear lens into how agriculture operates.

One of the participants determined he was going to select a grocery store as the influencer to target. He really struggled with identifying hot buttons while we were in the training and had a tendency to skew toward farm talk when I challenged him how to translate agriculture to a retailer.

The farmer wasn't feeling very confident when he left, but he pursued his personal action plan to connect with a grocery store in western Iowa where he lived. When he went home, he was so successful at asking questions, identifying retailer hot buttons, and translating agriculture for the grocers that he was able to create an ag day at the store. He and the grocer worked together to create an event that reached their mutual hot buttons of getting more consumers at the store, building their knowledge of food, and being positioned as good citizens in the community. That's a win-win-win. Grocer, farmer, and consumer all came out ahead!

You may not have spent a lot of time talking to people about what they're looking for in a grocery store. Please consider doing just that if you select retailers, moms, dads, or consumers as the group of influencers you'd like to engage in a conversation. If you catch someone with enough time to chat, you'll be able to ask questions, find hot buttons, and engage in a meaningful conversation.

Common interests in New York City

In another outreach effort, Laura Nelson had an opportunity to spend her day in conversation about food and farming in New York City. She describes herself as a writer, farm girl, amateur photographer, agvocate, cook, red dirt and classic rock music junkie, and egalitarian (it's a personal choice). Laura grew up on a diversified crop farm and cattle ranch on the Wyoming/Nebraska border and is now the editor of a newspaper in Montana. Look for the hot buttons and how she translated agriculture—beef in this case—to New Yorkers.

When you're passionate about being an agvocate, it's easy to get bogged down in negative news about our industry. We monitor vegan ballot initiatives, watch atrocious caught-in-the-act videos, and respond to soapbox-preaching food bloggers.

All noble causes, but also ones that can leave us feeling like it's "us" versus "them": ag versus consumers. I got a great reminder of this when I traveled to the Big Apple to work sampling Certified Angus Beef® steak to New Yorkers. I was prepared for some really tough con-

ROTTEN VEGETABLE 10
So often, we think we must educate people about farming. ("We have to educate consumers where their food comes from. We have educate them to thank farmers!") Wrong! Consider this: A salesperson walks into your office, sticks a finger right in your face, and says, "Let me educate you." You wouldn't like it any more than those we feel have to educate. How about we engage in a conversation—a two-way street—and learn as much as we try to teach? It's better than coming off as arrogant and narrow-minded!

sumer questions: hormones, CAFOs, animal welfare, beef nutrition, antibiotics, etc.

Instead of reciting sound bite after sound bite in defense of the beef industry, I re-discovered how much people love great steak and a simple story. People would casually grab a sample as they walked by, stop dead in their tracks to oooooh and ahhhhhh, then walk back to our booth and say, "That was the best steak I've ever had!"

I learned that New Yorkers don't typically have yards, so it's frivolous to share grilling tips. Some folks weren't familiar with the "tenderloin" cut. New Yorkers eat out a lot, and restaurant menus call it Filet Mignon. Being in New York doesn't mean you're a New Yorker... the city attracts a lot of tourists (duh!) from many places, backgrounds, and culinary tastes.

A quality product attracts a captive audience. But a captive audience doesn't mean an open door for a sales pitch. Rather, a good opportunity to visit with that person about a common interest—great steak, in my case!

Learning these things changed the course of my conversations, allowing me to better connect with our audience. I could share my message: Certified Angus Beef® is some of the best beef you can buy, raised by caring, dedicated Angus ranchers across America. The product quality is all about its marbling; look for our logo to make sure you're consistently getting the best.

That was my story, but each time I told it in a different way that met the needs and expectations of that individual.

Of course, to my dismay, each person I interacted with couldn't be an avid beef—loving carnivore! I heard several "No thanks, I'm not a big meat eater..." Not a good time to get defensive, regardless of the sinking feeling that brought on. Which reminds me: Isn't it strange how personal we can take someone's food choices?

It is personal to them, but we shouldn't take it that way. In a way, it's just a choice like the ones we make every day: paper or plastic, Deere or Case, iPhone or Blackberry, country music or rock, red meat or veggies, horse or ATV, pork or chicken, etc.

Like the Pat Green song says, "I guess we've all got our reasons." Trying to understand the reasoning behind another person's choice is the only way to empathize and relate. In my opinion, that's the only way to influence those choices.

For example, a question I got several times was: "Is this beef grass-fed?" Keep in mind, that's not an instant attack on grain-fed beef; it's an innocent question.

My answer would be something like this: "Of course it is—nearly all beef cattle are grass-fed for a large percentage of their lives. But to get the kind of marbling and flavor our customers like, the beef cattle that meet our standards are fed grain in the mature stages of their lives. Do you usually purchase grass-fed beef? Why is that? Can you taste a flavor difference?"

Those questions at the end are the keys. Trust me; you'll get further listening than talking, especially when you don't yet have a captive audience like I did.

I know most of you don't have an opportunity to initiate one-on-one conversations with New Yorkers who are enticed by the sights and smells of delicious steak samples. I had an unfair advantage.

But one advantage stays the same: a quality product and a quality story provides opportunity to change opinions. As agriculturalists, each of us should have a quality story to tell. If you don't, it's time to reevaluate what's happening on the ranch. I interviewed a feedlot manager once who told me, "We don't do anything here that we wouldn't be proud to have videotaped and shown to the world."

If you operate every day with that mentality, you have a quality product. So here's a refresher on sharing that story:

1. Focus on the audience you have. For those in animal agriculture, that's about 95% of the human population who enjoy an omnivorous diet just like you.

2. Capture that audience with a quality product and a quality story. Never miss an opportunity to make them feel good about your product. They'll hold it against your reputation every time your message or story isn't portrayed with the utmost quality.

3. Share that story on their terms. Memorized sound bites don't work. Molding those sound bites with empathy to ways that relate to another human's needs and interests do. Hot buttons are important.

4.   *Listen more than you talk, especially with an audience you haven't captivated yet. You're not selling anything; you're sharing information, and that's a two—way street.*

*You may think you have no hope of speaking the same language as urbanites. But they likely have interests such as hunting, family, sports, or cooking. **We are all human, and all of us have hot buttons.** Your job is to find common interests so you go from alien farmer to Joe the family man who has great grilling tips.*

You can easily do that by developing your own action plan and using the six steps to building a story. You don't need to be in a retail environment—try schools, local service organizations, or engaging in an online community. You never know where it will lead you!

Sassy grass farmer connects with politicians

Moving to the opposite coast, where issues on environmentalism are known to run strong, we meet Marie Bowers, a grass seed farmer in Oregon. Marie loves politics, fun shoes, and having a good time with her friends. She's also a spark plug known for making things happen, which has led her to various leadership roles in agricultural organizations such as American Agri-Women.

As you can imagine, farming in Oregon comes with its share of political challenges. Marie approaches this with a sassy smile and puts an action plan in place.

Everyone remembers the farm. The farm they grew up on, their grandparents had, or they visited as a child.

Politicians love to tell you about their "time" on the farm and any knowledge they have about farming. This stood out in my mind when talking to a female legislator about a bill in Oregon. She could care less that my dad was in the room, because she wanted to compare female farming adventures. Our commonality opened up a conversation to the issue at hand. She was empathetic to our cause because she remembered her own family's challenges.

Farms have changed drastically in their day-to-day operations over the past few decades. This scares people. They understood the importance of the farm they remember and realize the farm still holds a vital roll today. Connecting the changes from yesterday to today is key. Showing them that even the farm of yesteryear made progress and changes to remain viable just as the farm of today does.

Politicians are just people. They face the same challenge as the rest of us, dealing with the fact we are all human. I find knowing what they care about and asking questions goes a long ways to how receptive they are towards me.

Working with elected officials is about finding the common ground. No one hates the farmer, and most want farms to be successful. Sometimes they just need to reminisce and converse about the memory they have in order to understand your position.

I recall meeting with a state legislator who wanted a natural gas pipeline to go through his district. He was upset that the opposition came from groups and people who weren't his constituents but felt the need to oppose it. It was very easy to understand where he was coming from since we were there to talk about a similar situation. People and groups wanted to ban our agriculture practice of field burning, which is essential to the health of our fields. Most of the opposition were not directly affected by our activity. We were able to communicate about a bigger—picture issue in society and then translate those concerns to our own issues.

In reality, most agricultural issues we face result in a bigger fundamental issue within society. We just need to realize they are human, know their key issues (hot buttons) and then leverage those hot buttons to connect agriculture.

If you are like most farmers, you don't know a whole lot about growing grass seed, except for wanting to eradicate it from your fields. Marie gives you a glimpse into that world at her blog, http://oregongreen.wordpress.com.

60-year-old finds real connections through social media

Remember Larry Sailer, the 60-year-old corn, bean and hog farmer in Iowa from Chapter 1? He says, "Social media has kept me from being a cranky old pig farmer!" Larry has been on CNN and Reuters and has hosted a Japanese television crew because of his activity through social media. Not what you'd expect for a shy old hog farmer who was once terrified of speaking in front of others!

Just in the last four years, an amazing transformation has occurred. I always strive to do a better job of sharing my story. At a Farm Bureau meeting, I was introduced to Facebook and Twitter. I did ask one of my kids and grandkids to set me up "online" but have become much more comfortable.

Part of my motivation was that I had met several people around the country that I thought I could keep in touch with by using this new technology. Just imagine an old hog farmer on his iPad and smart phone.

The first year, Facebook did a good job keeping me in touch with my friends to share ideas and encourage each other. Then I attended the first AgChat Foundation in Chicago. The group of farmers and ag folks who put the Foundation together somehow had the vision to see the power of these new tools to connect with people that were newly searching for answers to how and where their food is produced.

I learned how to communicate with the world. This has connected me to people I can learn from, and to be able to share with them my thoughts.

Social media has opened doors that I did not even know were there. It has also let people see into my operation. Most farmers are not trying to hide what they do. They are just very private.

*This can get very uncomfortable. **But we must be transparent to be believable.***

I have had interviews that made me look bad, but I have also been able to share who I am and what I do.

A live spot on CNN even propelled me into sharing my farm through a blog. Even though I did not blog at the time, somehow they thought I was a farming blogger because the other three people on the panel were. This is something I have tried to use. They acted like they had seen a ghost. Here I was, a sixty-year-old hog farmer that writes a blog and uses Facebook and Twitter.

Shortly after that, just by chance, I chatted with Shannon Latham, a young mother supporting the Franklin County 4-H Foundation. I learned she has a degree in journalism and she agreed to let me guest blog on her blog every Tuesday at thefieldpostion.com. Shannon takes my random thoughts and ideas and makes them readable.

This has given me a presence on the Internet that can be googled (now that's a term I could not have imagined back when I started to farm). I have been found by TV crews and reporters from as far away as Japan. Not bad for a shy old hog farmer from Franklin County, Iowa.

Much of the social media landscape has to do with mindset, not age, as Larry illustrates. Opportunities abound to create conversation around farm and food, whether on camera, in person, or online.

A recent Center for Food Integrity (CFI) research report illustrates the disconnect between farm and fork.[47] Let's use the findings as a backdrop to challenge you to consider how you would answer four questions to grow the conversation.

- Only 1 in 5 believes today's food supply is safer than when they were growing up. **How can you tell your story to help people understand how important this is to you and what practices have been put in place that have improved food safety?.**
- 1 in 4 strongly believe animals are treated humanely (down from 1 in 3 in the prior year's study). **How does this feel to you, and where can you illustrate how much of a priority animal care is?**
- Food prices are a great concern to 53%, and only 30% strongly agree that US food is amongst the most affordable in the world today. **How have you worked to keep food prices down, and where are you seeing the increases coming from?**
- 40% don't believe the United States has a responsibility to provide food to the rest of the world; 53% would rather teach people in other countries how to feed themselves. **Why does feeding the world matter to you?**

Those numbers are a bit of a reality check, aren't they? They offer a wake-up call about the importance of bridging the divide(s) across the food plate. *No More Food Fights!* is full of real-life examples on how to put an action plan in place and make it work—and you'll see people doing just that on the food side of the book if you read it, but keep in mind that you are the linchpin in all of this.

You! Put Your Own Passion to Work

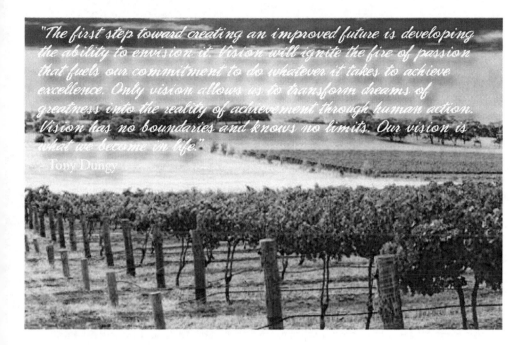

"The first step toward creating an improved future is developing the ability to envision it. Vision will ignite the fire of passion that fuels our commitment to do whatever it takes to achieve excellence. Only vision allows us to transform dreams of greatness into the reality of achievement through human action. Vision has no boundaries and knows no limits. Our vision is what we become in life."
~ Tony Dungy

D o you have the passion to pursue a vision of a connected food plate, in which conversation flows back and forth? Do you have the passion to reach out your hand when you're in uncomfortable discussions about farming, ask questions, and then learn? Do you have the vision to move agriculture forward?

This half step is labeled as such because I wanted it to stand out as the most important. **Your passion is the fuel you'll need for an ongoing, consistent discussion about our business.**

Is true leadership about me or we?

Few are intuitive leaders moving through life with the masses following them. Most of us have to learn leadership. It's always interesting in my work with agricultural advocates to watch them go from succeeding individually to learning to bring others along in the agvocacy journey. More than once, I've had the conversation with people who

---

CONNECTION POINT 12
Do you need resources to be proactive in talking about ag? See my Agriculture & Food Resources Page at http://www.causematters. com/ag-resources/for a wealth of blogs links, advocacy tips, and background information.

have succeeded as individuals, "This is no longer about you but the bigger picture. Your work is to now create more advocates like you."

Only the best become true leaders. Many get distracted by ego, politics, or the latest bright, shiny object. When I see leaders rising through the ranks, I start watching to see if they'll be able

ROTTEN VEGETABLE 11
Promoting your position exclusively. Some groups find it necessary to continually grandstand. There is no single answer in the discussion about food. Why not learn about other positions and even share those perspectives with others for a more well-rounded discussion?

to make the jump from "me" to "we." As a professional speaker training people in advocacy, I'm fortunate to witness many of these journeys; when people transition to the "we" of agriculture, it is my single greatest motivator.

Olympian finds farmer to be a blurred image

Inspiring others in a shared vision can be a massive undertaking, particularly when you're training for an international competition, yet some people can do it well. One of those people. is Garrett Weber-Gale.

Helping people be healthier through what they eat has become Garrett's mission in life. Quite an undertaking for a guy carrying around two Olympic medals and who has shared the podium with Michael Phelps and is training for the World Championships. He knows what he puts into his body is the direct fuel he gets out and has realized food is a priority.

Interestingly, Garrett's passion for using food to be healthier and for inspiring others to do so began when he was diagnosed with dangerously high blood pressure at the age of 19. He was forced to radically change his diet and take medications. Three years later, he brought home two gold medals.[48]

I've not talked to many Olympians but was surprised to find that Garrett's sport doesn't define him. He's just as excited about his future, which revolves around food and nutrition. He's developed cooking techniques based on classic recipes and techniques he learned in some of the top kitchens around the world. Garrett has plans to write a book about how healthy food doesn't have to taste bad; open a fast-food restaurant offering delicious, healthy food; and inspire others to be healthier through what they put in their bodies as a part of Athletic Foodie™at www.Athletic Foodie.com.

Garrett's food choices include fresh produce, grains, legumes, red meat one or two times per week, and poultry/egg/fish once per week. He prefers to eat seasonally, buy organic, and shop at the farmer's market close to where he lives in Austin, Texas. He likes to shop the outside of the grocery story and avoid the aisles, as whole foods in their natural state are a priority. He loves tasty food—especially when it's good for you.

Garrett's views seem fairly mainstream to me; he's read some of Michael Pollan's work (author of *The Omnivore's Dilemma* and *Food Rules* and contributor to the movie Food, Inc.) but is familiar with the volatility involved with farming. When I asked him what comes to mind when he thinks of a farmer, he indicated that a farmer is now a blurred image. He grew up in Wisconsin, knew people who had farms, and thought of them working day and night to try to grow food.

He is concerned that much of what we eat is from farms with higher rates of production. He

> **ROTTEN VEGETABLE 12**
> Practicing strong ethics and living a life of integrity should be unspoken requirements in any business or household. Today's environment makes it easy to try to stretch the truth just a bit. Don't give in to the temptation. You'll be respected more in the end for having the guts to say no.

remembers farms as being on "much smaller plots of land" in Wisconsin and also remembers picking apples at his local apple orchard, so seeing apples from New Zealand in the grocery makes no sense to him.

When asked where he finds information about food and nutrition, Garrett is quick to point to places from websites to Twitter to the *New York Times* to the *Huffington Post*. He enjoys talking to people about nutrition but suggests governmental websites, RDs, people in the field, agricultural sites, chefs, and nutritional books for finding food insight. Note the predominant online influence, which is consistent with findings from the Center for Food Integrity that show websites as people's main source for information about food.[49]

Garrett also mentioned that his teammates haven't been to a farm and that most people are so detached from farms that they don't think about where their food comes from. Some of his questions for farmers are:

- *What are you growing? Why?*
- *What did you grow 10, 20, 30 years ago?*
- *Are you happy with where you sell?*
- *Who controls your price?*
- *How much depends on market, price, supply, and demand?*
- *What do you need to continue progressing?*
- *What are you eating?*

Think about those questions as you connect with the mainstream. You may not agree with Garrett, but I think you can learn a great deal from his food choices and influences. I found commonalities with Garrett in my belief that healthy food can taste good, though I'm not going to pretend to eat nearly as healthily as a world-class athlete. One of the last questions I asked him was how to engage in a civil conversation. **"People usually go into a conversation with preconceived ideology. Be open to everyone's viewpoint,"** he replied. On that, we absolutely agree!

Passion can both attract and push others away. You'll likely find many more hands to shake if you approach the food plate with the willingness to listen and learn. This will also help others learn.

Can agriculture lead into the future?

Let's pause to consider what is taught children who grow up on farms and ranches. Creativity to solve whatever problem comes up, strong work ethic, honesty, and perseverance are great farm-kid traits. At some level, so are the independent mindset, stubbornness, and modesty that are prevalent in agriculture. But is that what we really want to be passing on to the next generation?

Don't get me wrong; my farm roots trace back several generations, so I know those traits are ingrained in agriculture's culture. I'll also fully own that I'm as stubborn as a mule and rather hardheaded, but working with people around all sides of the food plate makes me wonder if those are the skills we need to lead in agriculture's future.

I see farmers and ranchers who care deeply about bringing a voice to agriculture but who can't work together because of being so independently minded. This is true in policy discussions, in the most well-intended efforts to connect with consumers, and as new groups are forming to benefit the big picture of agriculture. Perhaps you'll want to throw rotten vegetables and cow pies at me, but I have to ask the tough questions to people across all sectors of agriculture.

Why is it so easy for agriculture to be divided and conquered, as with the HSUS, organic versus conventional, and food versus fuel? Why do people, for example, feel the need to line up behind the Grocery Manufacturer's Association **or** corn folks? There is more than enough corn to go around. Sure, feed prices stink for those who have animals. As a dairy person, I get that! But were the corn and soybean growers squawking when beef, milk, chicken, and pork producers were making a decent profit?

Let me suggest this: count to 50 and tap your boots together three times before you publicly condemn another part of agriculture, because in the long-haul, this will likely impact *your* success. I'd strongly encourage you to hold your national organizations to the same standards. This is true whether you're talking, tweeting, or Facebooking—know that you are agriculture to those outside of our business.

Do farmers and ranchers care enough to speak out proactively? It's easy to respond to the nasty videos, to get up in arms about defending your favorite piece of legislation, or to promote a group you're affiliated with. It's a lot tougher to take the risk of reaching across the food plate, whether it's having a conversation with an extended family member or engaging in a Twitter debate, going to your local economic development meeting or writing a blog. I've worked in agricultural advocacy for more than a decade and have to ask whether we care enough to truly listen and seek ways to engage proactively. Every day. Or can we only respond?

Is our window so narrow that we sometimes lose sight of the big picture? Frankly, the microclimate affecting a ranch in California or the nuances of a small meat processor in Ohio aren't of great concern to the people we are trying to connect with. The well-being of the *big* picture of agriculture is—especially as it affects them as food buyers. I understand you have to worry about your own business and family first, but shouldn't we all be responsible for taking the blinders off a bit more and

<u>focusing on the big picture</u> rather than only looking at our own small piece of the ag world?

Why is it OK to text a photo of your new combine but not to talk to a reporter or update your Facebook? Studies have clearly shown that mainstream media doesn't have access to enough expert sources to food and agriculture. You don't have to have all the answers, but know that the media will find information—and it may just be from Greenpeace or the HSUS.

If you want the story told truthfully, it's time to push modesty, stubborness and fear aside. While you're at it, please take a couple of minutes to put that picture on Facebook with a note about why it's so cool so those outside the farm world can gain perspective.

Not everyone will agree with or like what I've written here. That's okay. If I've inspired some thought, incited discussion, or caused action—my mission has been accomplished.

Actions speak louder than words. Are you sure your actions are best serving agriculture's future?

CHAPTER 7

Build an Action Plan to
Help You Reach Across the Plate

"If you want a year of prosperity, grow grain. If you want a decade of prosperity, grow trees. If you want a century of prosperity, grow people."
– Chinese Proverb

F unny how we spend so much time thinking about the technical side of agriculture, isn't it? The people side of the business will ultimately determine our success—whether on a farm, on a ranch, in agribusiness, or as part of an ag organization. How can you put some elbow grease into an action plan to help grow people?

Create your own action plan for meaningful conversations

1.   **Who** do you need to develop a relationship with? Focus on **specific influencer groups**.

Influencer group   Goal for conversation

_____   _____

_____   _____

_____   _____

2. **What** are their **hot buttons**? Remember, hot buttons don't need to be about food or farming!

      Influencer group   Hot buttons

      _____   _____

      _____   _____

      _____   _____

3. **Why** should agriculture matter to them? **Speak their language** through their hot buttons, not through ag or farm talk!

      Hot buttons   Messages to connect food and farming

      _____   _____

      _____   _____

      _____   _____

4. **Where** will you be reaching across the plate? Think about **places or tools** you are most likely to find your key influencer group interested in a conversation.

      Influencer group   Where to best connect

      _____   _____

      _____   _____

      _____   _____

5. **When** will you build this bridge; what's your **time line**?

      Influencer group   Expected time line

      _____   _____

      _____   _____

      _____   _____

6. **How** is this going to matter to the **big picture** of agriculture and step 6 ½, connect with **your passion**?

      _____   _____

      _____   _____

      _____   _____

Michael Pollan penned, "I very much like to have a personal stake in what I'm writing about." This conversation is deeply personal for me; farming is woven into the fabric of who I am, as it likely is for you. It's not something we've wrote about in the journalism department at an Ivy League school; it's what we've lived.

If you believe agriculture needs a stronger voice for agriculture from those with their hands in the soil, I challenge you to move the conversation to a different level. <u>Now</u>, not tomorrow.

I hope the 6 1/2 steps to a more meaningful conversation about food and farming will help you share the story of agriculture with others as you reach across the food plate. After all, if you're not reaching across the plate, who is speaking for you?

Let's meet in the middle. It's a much nicer place—and smells a lot better—than a food fight.

CHAPTER 8

Can You Connect at the Center of the Plate?

"My own experience is to use the tools that are out there. Use the digital world. But never lose sight of the need to reach out and talk to other people who don't share your view. Listen to them and see if you can find a way to compromise."
~ Colin Powell

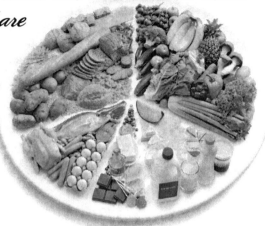

Take a look at the plate at the beginning of this chapter. What do you see? A plethora of food? A need for lower food prices? Amazingly diverse products? Nutritional expertise or obesity epidemic? Brilliant advances or industrial problems? Nutrition for everyone or for only the privileged?

What do you feel when you look at the food plate? Disgust? Hunger? Curious about why your portion of the plate isn't bigger? Gratitude that the United States and Canada (and most developed countries) have this type of plate available regularly? Confusion about what you're supposed to be doing when you go to the grocery store?

ROTTEN VEGETABLE 13
Is your passion driving others away? Are you so outspoken that people only hear you screaming? Passionate agriculture and food people attract others like bees to honey. Sure, some can be passionate naysayers, but it's a small percentage. Why not find common points in your passion to get excited about farming and food together? Hint: this means you have to rein your passion in enough to listen to each other.

When I look at the plate, I see people with tremendous expertise around all sides of it. Chefs who marry many food flavors, farmers who grow crops and animals, processors who clean and package food, registered dietitians who help us know the best nutrition for our well-being, and many more.

Yet, I also see dividing lines, which frustrates me—as you could tell on the food side of the book with the trip around the grocery store that left me with a headache and a sore tongue. Meat versus vegetables. Dairy versus soy. Small versus large. Organic versus conventional. Corn versus sugar. One label versus another.

The point of *No More Food Fights!* is to encourage a civil conversation; it's about **people working together to understand the many perspectives around the plate.** I'd like to look at that same plate and see polarized conversations move toward the middle.

Compromise can be viewed as a dirty word—some seem to think it means they have to give up their own point of view. Look at it as bringing your own perspective and then adding more ideas to enrich the conversation. The same could be said with meeting in the middle. It's not a political statement in *No More Food Fights!*, but a visual of where we can go to shake hands.

After all, the conversation becomes rather lopsided—and self-serving—causing the plate to go off kilter if it's farm versus food. That's when the food fights begin and can stink up the place. But we can find balance if we meet in the middle.

CONNECTION POINT 13

How do you politely disengage from those not interested in a courteous conversation? My estimate is that 10% on either side of the spectrum (entrenched or inflamed) aren't interested in a lot more than promoting their positions. I suggest that removing the platform from grandstanders takes away their stage, which takes energy from their cause. You do so by thanking them for their time, then walking away—and being disciplined enough to not get into a negative or competitive debate.

Instead, focus on those you can engage in a productive conversation. Productive doesn't equal agreement, but it does equal meaning. Look for common values, human interest, hot buttons. Start there, rather than trying to tackle the major issues first. Each person around the food plate is human, with human interests.

Who can lead the conversation to the center?

"Thought leadership" is a term thrown around a fair amount in the business environment. It may be considered cliché by some or, as I've found, make most people scratch their heads. If you have the ability to approach a subject with perspective on both sides of the issue, you are a thought leader. These are key leadership elements that bridge the gap and bring people to the center of the plate:

- **Passion.** It acts as a magnet. It propels a movement. It engages a community. Thought leaders have the ability to channel their passion for the good of the greater cause.

64   No More Food Fights!

- **Honesty.** It's easy to pretend to be someone else in today's social media—driven society, and some people thrive on building false profiles. Don't be anyone but you!

- **Ears.** Can you hear a question from across the food plate and really *listen?* Do you automatically go into defense mode? Are you coming up with your answer while the other person is talking? Thought leaders ask others questions and listen closely to the answers.

- **Guts enough to accept change**—and, preferably, embrace it. You're as young as you're ever going to be today—are you really sure you want to spend your life complaining about change? Many reference their ages for not understanding social media, but I've seen 65-year-old grandpas outpace 25-year-old guys in using Facebook. Don't let your birthdate, position, or embarrassment prevent you from adapting to change!

- **Big picture**. Thinking long-term and looking beyond your own business to understand global demands is essential to leading the food and farm conversation. This provides consideration of the impact of policy, activism and markets influencing the big picture conversation.

- **Curiosity.** Children thrive on it; adults bury it. Sometimes, the simple act of asking why can lead you down an entirely different path. Curiosity is an element of leadership that will help you discern what's important to the people you're trying to talk to about food and farm.

- **Execution.** If you don't have the ability to put wheels under ideas and involve others in pulling the wagon, you'll be stuck. Bright shiny objects are fun, but they become dull over time and get put away in the back of the closet. Only those who can execute, stay focused, and grow ideas are true leaders.

- **Open mind.** Many think our greatest days of innovation are in the past. I disagree; the food-and-farm discussion is a frontier desperately in need of thought leadership. Look at the technologies, businesses, communities, and techniques available to you now that didn't exist five years ago. Be open enough to find a way to adapt them for the benefit of the big picture.

- **Tenacity for the long haul.** Few parts of agriculture or food can be called easy business. Agendas around a myriad of issues, often fueled by misinformation, add to the challenge, but always know that one voice, a single picture, or a tweet may just capture the attention of thousands and make people stop to consider the middle of the plate.

- **Humility** enough to admit when you're wrong and to apologize when needed. There's not a better teacher of this than parenthood. Everyone makes mistakes; own up to them and move on. Humility is rare in those holding leadership positions, but the few who possess it can lead a movement as servant—leaders.

- **Optimism**. If you don't believe in a better tomorrow, why bother?

- **Willingness to have the tough conversations.** Is local and organic better? Do we still need subsidies? Why are your farming/cooking practices better or worse than mine? Do food buyers have a right to demand labels? Are animals living in better conditions? This is difficult, but thought leadership is about leading the conversation, not reacting to it. It's also about taking the high road even when others sink to the gutter.

Truthfully, I'd like to see more thought leadership in the food and farming conversation. We all sing to the choir that we have to do things differently, so how about we actually put some muscle where our mouths are?

Putting your fork, knife, spoon, and knife to work

Silverware can help with that. Let's take a look at how we can put the fork, spoon, and knife to work in reaching across the plate. Please note: this is reaching—not poking or hitting. Play nice with your silverware.

Fork: Connecting tines

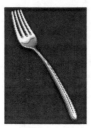

The fork is perhaps the most commonly used utensil in the Western world. It can be used for stabbing, swiping, and scooping food. It can also stick people in the back—as those people who want to throw smelly rotten tomatoes in a food fight seem to do through grandstanding and positioning.

To me, the fork represents a stake in the ground. On one side of the plate, you have the pitchfork. Hopefully you realize by now that modernization has eliminated many pitchforks and farmers don't look like the *American Gothic* farmer portrait, but we're going with a pitchfork as a visual example. These forks are busily at work worrying about what needs to happen on the farm. On the other side, you have the dining fork concerned about feeding a family the best food possible—with conflicting needs depending on socioeconomic status and geography.

Is it possible for those forks to become more similar in their interests? Yes, if both sides pause and look around to see where the commonalities are. After all, we are all humans. Most have an interest in family, sports, school, community, national well-being, eating, friends, and the like. Don't let people around you raise their forks in fear of the conversation; what would happen if the tines connected? A bridge would be formed.

Spoon: Warming the relationship

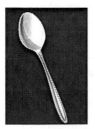

Pour some sugar on me! Yes, I'm a rock 'n' roll fan, but spoons have such a happy feel to them. Whether you're sipping soup, hanging them from your nose, or eating ice cream, the spoon is a utensil that's not only practical but also warming.

What if we applied that same idea to the conversation around the food plate? I'm not suggesting you spoon with the person you're connecting with around the food plate (bodily spooning would likely create more than food fights!), but I do believe we can easily have a practical discussion. As people find value in the conversation—and an understanding about their particular positions—there will be a warming to the relationship that leads to trust.

Ultimately, that's what brings people to the center of the plate—respect and trust—even when there is not 100% agreement. Remember the spoon to help you warm a relationship.

Knife: Leveraging a community

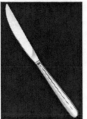

The Transportation Security Administration (TSA) considers the knife a dangerous weapon, and most of you probably have negative images of knives going into skin. Let's look at it in a different light. Imagine this: a few peas placed on the end of the knife, slightly bent back, aimed at the person across the table from you. It's kind of fun to imagine that kind of leveraging, isn't it?

Rather than flinging food, consider the leveraging power knives can have in lifting and moving items. Leveraging is critical in this discussion. Don't just reach your hand across—find others to join you in getting to know people across the table.

In other words, leverage a community to build a movement. After watching thousands of people from around the world connect virtually through communities such as AgChat and FoodChat, I know firsthand the power in building communities that leverage the passions people have about food and farming.

The greatest power we have in this is a combined interest in food and farming. Think of the knife to help you leverage that!

Looking for exact answers in how to have a meaningful conversation? Take a look at the utensils around the plate, and consider how the fork, spoon, and knife can help build connections. Then take a look at the person holding the silverware.

Do you have enough guts to meet in the middle?

True leadership is influence—not only influence within a small circle, but grasping—and in turn influencing—the bigger picture. The conversation around food and farm is in desperate need of those leaders, not of someone who can simply tell his or her story and string a line of manure. Not the most gifted at debate. And certainly not a dictator who sees his or her opinion as the answer for all.

The most effective leaders I've seen combine passion with human-ness, which makes them effective in connecting with others. **Consider the middle of the food plate; it's where hands meet in a handshake, trust is built, and human connections form.**

Thought leadership around the food plate will lead people to the middle—and requires authenticity, a bit of audacity, and a whole lot of action.

Authenticity. Keep it real. What if you were asked to engage in a conversation with 10 people holding different viewpoints about food? It helps to acknowledge that your part of the plate doesn't always get it right, though you try your best.

As discussed throughout this book, neither side of the plate has done the best job at connecting. Don't let food become the next religion and politics—have an open conversation.

Audacity. This is having guts enough to do what needs to be done. To put it in farm terms, will you be the bull or the steer? I'm not suggesting we charge anyone and knock down gates, but perhaps we should be a bit more aggressive in seeking ways to connect—especially in times when there is no war to fight.

In other words, be audacious enough to be proactive—not in a bold, arrogant way, but with enough gumption to try something new, whether it's going beyond the choir or trying out new media.

Action. Are you an active or reactive leader? Leaders don't wait until the rotten veggies are thrown by the other side, because they understand the trust of the middle is being eroded.

Action as a leader in today's hyperconnected world must include the ability to gather and engage the 80% of people who can still be influenced. This action is required in times of response *and* status quo. Meeting in the middle should be a proactive daily occurrence, not a response mechanism.

If you're passionate about any part of the conversation connecting gate to plate, here's my challenge to you: **Authentically consider what you want to accomplish, be audacious enough to try new ideas, and take action to bring others to the table.** In other words, know what your goal is, have the guts to pursue it, and surround yourself with the best people who believe in the cause.

Many have suggested I include screen shots of the grandstanding happening online, examples of conversations gone awry, and specific outlines of what the right kind of conversation looks like in *No More Food Fights!* I'm not doing that because stories interwoven through the 6 ½ steps for the ag folks and the six senses for the food folks are the best examples I can offer.

As I finished writing this book, a great quote from executive coach Scott Eblin popped up in my e-mail: "Keeping people informed keeps them calm."

What is the unique perspective you bring to the table? How are you informing people about your side of the food plate? If each person collectively brings his or her information to the table, I hope we can have the majority of people at the table be calm—and be civil—in our conversation.

Take a look 20 years down the road. What does the food plate look like? Will it be painted by people with authenticity, audacity, and action—or rhetoric? If you think food and farming have changed in the past two decades, be prepared for even greater change—and a greater disconnect.

My single wish? *No More Food Fights!* has made you think about how to grow your conversation about food and farm. You decide who has the vision to make the boldest strokes in reaching across the plate; those will be the people painting the food plate of the future. **I believe we have the opportunity to re-write tomorrow's history of farm and food.**

Actions to connect at the center of the plate are the same whether you're on the farm or food side. If you flip the book over and read the other side, you'll see this final chapter is identical. That's because reaching across the plate to shake hands looks the same, no matter what angle you approach it from. Are you willing to grow that connection into a more meaningful conversation about food and farm?

References

36 Maslansky Luntz + Partners. US Farmers and Ranchers Research Roadmap. October 2012. Research can be requested from USFRA or the author by contacting info@fooddialogues.com or 636-449-5086.

37 Tardanico, Susan. "How to Make People Glad to See You: Advice From a Legend." *Forbes.* June 2012. http://www.forbes.com/sites/susantardanico/2012/06/26/how-to-make-people-glad-to-see-you-advice-from-a-legend/

38 CharlieArnot. Center for Food Integrity. Journal of Rural Sociology. December 2009.

39 Chipotle. "Back to the Start." *YouTube.* August 2011. http://www.youtube.com/watch?v=aMfSGt6rHos

40 Webster, Maeve. "Perception versus Reality: A Food Study." *Charleston | Orwig.* October 2012. http://charlestonorwig.com/2012Event/perception.aspx

41 "Building Healthy America: A Profile of the Supplemental Nutrition Assistance Program." *USDA.* April 2012. http://www.fns.usda.gov/ora/MENU/Published/snap/FILES/Other/BuildingHealthyAmerica.pdf

42 "Building Healthy America: A Profile of the Supplemental Nutrition Assistance Program." *USDA.* April 2012. http://www.fns.usda.gov/ora/MENU/Published/snap/FILES/Other/BuildingHealthyAmerica.pdf

43 "Building Healthy America: A Profile of the Supplemental Nutrition Assistance Program." *USDA.* April 2012. http://www.fns.usda.gov/ora/MENU/Published/snap/FILES/Other/BuildingHealthyAmerica.pdf

44 "Know Your Farmer, Know Your Food." *USDA.* http://www.usda.gov/wps/portal/usda/knowyourfarmer?navid=KNOWYOURFARMER

45 Miller, Marlys. "What Do Consumers Think of Today's Farmers?" *Pork Network.* November 2011. http://www.porknetwork.com/pork-news/-What-do-consumers-think-of-todays-farmers-134135798.html

46 Nestle, Marion. "Surprise! Consumers Don't Trust the Meat Industry." *Food Politics.* October 2011. http://www.foodpolitics.com/2011/10/surprise-consumers-dont-trust-the-meat-industry/

47 "Top Things You Should Know from Research of the Issues Webinar." *Center for Food Integrity.* November 2012. Request copy at http://www.foodintegrity.org/research.

[49] D'Amato, Gary. "Former Olympian Weber-Gale to Speak at UWM." *Journal Sentinel Online*. October 2012. http://www.jsonline.com/sports/etc/former-olympian-webergale-to-speak-at-uwm-49759bu-173222451.html

[49] Muirhead, Sarah. "Study Shows Shift in Food Information Source." *Feedstuffs*. May 2011. http://www.feedstuffs.com/ME2/dirmod.asp?sid=&nm=&type=Publishing&mod=Publications::Article&mid=AA01E1C62E954234AA0052ECD5818EF4&tier=4&id=7FE2C6472C7A4E3CB37F63F8AFD79D13

About the Author

A farm girl since birth and a foodie since eating in Italy, Michele Payn-Knoper is one of North America's leading farm and food advocates. She has helped thousands of people in agricultural, dietetic, and food audiences connect the farm gate to the food plate.

Michele wrote *No More Food Fights!* to encourage people around the food plate to connect in the interest of growing a more productive conversation. After all, food fights can be fun, but they usually end up stinking! She invites you to explore the different sides of the plate and to think about food a little differently as you make decisions for your family.

Michele has built farm and food connections in more than 25 countries and earned the Certified Speaking Professional designation awarded to less than 10% of professional speakers globally. She also founded AgChat and FoodChat, virtual communities connecting thousands of agriculture and food people—many of whom are featured in *No More Food Fights!* Michele is an in-demand media resource whose work has been featured across agricultural media, on food panels, and in major media channels such as *USA Today* and *CNN* to translate firsthand farm experience to the 98.5% of the population not on a farm.

She has owned cattle and baked bread since she was nine years old, and she believes her life's calling is to connect those two worlds. Michele provides a framework for farmers, dietitians, chefs, food scientists, ranchers, consumers, agribusiness, and foodies to reach across the plate and shake hands. She holds BS degrees in animal science and agricultural communications from Michigan State University, where the story of her impact has been featured in a *Spartan Saga*.

Widely recognized for the passion and fire she brings to agriculture and nutrition organizations across the United States and Canada, Michele knows her best audience is in her family's kitchen and barn in west central Indiana. That's where food—and conversation—is to be appreciated, enjoyed, and even celebrated. She invites others to join her in the journey toward connecting farm and food.

MPK Wants to Hear From You!

Want to arrange for Michele to help your group grow the conversation around food and agriculture? Discover for yourself why she's known for lighting up a room, taking audiences on a roller coaster of emotions—and getting them kickboxing. Visit http://causematters.com for MPK's speaking programs and for her *Gate to Plate* blog.

Looking for connections happening around the food plate right now? Interested in resources for the international agriculture and dietetic communities? Check out MPK's Facebook page at http://facebook.com/causematters or follow @mpaynknoper on Twitter at http://twitter.com/mpaynknoper.

Ready to share a story about how you've seen growth in the farm-and-food conversation? Have a great example of people reaching across the plate? With your permission, Michele may feature your work as an example. E-mail your story to book@causematters.com.

In the meantime, keep reaching across the plate!

Use this QR code for
extras to help you
grow the conversation

Praise for *No More Food Fights!*

"There's no need to have food fights in the grocery aisles. *No More Food Fights!* provides a fresh look at some of the dilemmas food buyers and farmers both face. More importantly, this book gives ideas to get everyone around the food plate engaged in a conversation."

—Phil Lempert, The Supermarket Guru®,
NBC News' *Today* Show Food Trends Editor, Author, and Speaker

"*No More Food Fights!* takes a unique look at the very real problem of a disconnect between farm and food. Michele Payn-Knoper offers an intriguing look at tough issues such as food safety, animal welfare and biotechnology. We are delighted she brought food, nutrition and agriculture experts together."

—David Schmidt, President & CEO, International Food Information Council

"There is a natural connection between food and farm that's lost to most grocery shoppers. *No More Food Fights!* offers an inside look at some of the most critical issues that people around the food plate need to be talking about today."

—Janet Helm, MS, RD, author of *The Food Lover's Healthy Habits Cookbook*
and former media spokesperson for the Academy of Nutrition and Dietetics

"From acknowledging concerns and establishing shared values, to transparency and engagement, the topics addressed in Michele Payn-Knoper's *No More Food Fights!* offer a roadmap for today's ongoing national dialogue about food and farming. It all starts with listening and building trust and, at the end of the day, sharing personal stories rich in information so our customers can make informed decisions on their own and connect with farm and ranch families at the center of the plate."

—Bob Stallman, President, American Farm Bureau Federation

"When you understand where your food comes from, you can make better health decisions. I always recommend people ask the experts - and Michele Payn-Knoper is one of the best at bridging the farm and food worlds. *No More Food Fights!* is a much-needed resource that will give you a personal look at why getting the real dish about food matters."

—Eliz Greene, Wellness Expert and Speaker, American Heart Association Spokesperson

No More Food Fights! is the perfect antidote to daily servings of sensationalized misinformation about our food supply and agriculture practices. Since food is meant to be enjoyed and savored rather than feared, Michele Payn-Knoper nourishes you with practical advice and accurate answers from the experts. No portion control needed with this lively and inspiring guide - devour this book in entirety!

—Kim Galeaz, RD, CD, Registered Dietitian. Culinary Nutritionist. Recipe Creator, Writer and host of *Indiana Cooks* on WFYI

"Agriculture needs to address food buyer concerns in order to be successful in the future. Food buyers need to know more facts about where their food comes from. Michele Payn-Knoper bridges those worlds in *No More Food Fights!* and helps others do the same. A must-read."

—Mary Shelman, Harvard Business School Agribusiness Program

NO MORE FOOD FIGHTS!

GROWING A PRODUCTIVE
FARM AND FOOD CONVERSATION

Food fights might seem entertaining, but there's nothing funny about the fights taking place over food production. Resource limitations, animal welfare, and biotechnology are just a few issues cropping up to create confusion in the grocery store. Ultimately, both farmers and food buyers are making a personal choice, and author Michele Payn-Knoper calls for decorum instead of mayhem in the conversation around farm and food.

In an effort to break stereotypes, one side of this book describes farmers who don't wear overalls but who do use technology in producing food and preserving the environment, dairy farmers who work on "cow comfort," and how hard farmers work on sustainability. On the other side, the book reminds farmers that only a tiny percentage of the population lives on a farm and urges farmers to tell their stories through social media and everyday conversation to correct mistaken beliefs about food production perpetuated by traditional media.

The book's very design lends itself to exploring both sides of the issue. One side of *No More Food Fights!* is aimed at those who primarily consume food—chefs, healthcare professionals, foodies, dietitians, and retailers. Flipping the book reveals the other side, which is geared toward those who produce food—farmers, agricultural businesses, and ranchers.

Throughout the book, the author intersperses personal stories from farmers, food scientists, dietitians, and ranchers. She naturally guides readers from both sides to "reach across the plate" to honestly explore food concerns and the critical connection from farm gate to food plate. Bring peace to your plate—and your next trip to the grocery store—with *No More Food Fights!* as your guide.

Sincere appreciation to the photography talent found throughout this book. Photo credits belong to the following individuals:
    Food Chapters 3, 4, 6 and Farm Chapter 6: Joe Murphy
    Food Chapter 5, Food & Farm Introductions and Farm Chapter 1, 7: Emmert Photography
    Food Chapter 1, 7, and Farm Chapter 3: Lauren Chase, Montana Stockgrowers Association
    Farm Chapter 2: Renee Kelly
    Food Chapter 2: Zach and Anna Hunnicutt

Cover graphic by Kanaly Design

First published by Dog Ear Publishing
4010 W. 86th Street, Ste H
Indianapolis, IN 46268
www.dogearpublishing.net

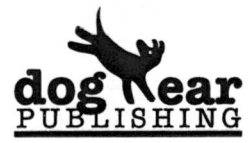

ISBN: 978-1-4575-1722-8

This book is printed on acid-free paper.

Printed in the United States of America

To my daughter, who serves as a daily inspiration to grow the conversation around food and farm. I hope you'll always love playing with cows and baking bread— and standing up for what you believe in.

Acknowledgements

"A life without cause is a life without effect."

~ Author unknown

Those words, on the wall above my desk, are a daily reminder of the power of serving a cause. An individual can't create effect without a community—I'd be remiss to not thank the many people my agricultural, food, and local communities.

More than 35 people from around the food plate contributed stories to this book and are recognized in the chapters, along with links so others can connect with these respected sources. I thank each person who allowed me to interview them, or provided their story in their own words. Your example added tremendous dimension to the discussion.

Talented photographers Joe Murphy, Lauren Chase of Montana Stockgrowers and Vicki Emmert graciously provided the beautiful photos at the beginning of each chapter. Thank you for bringing visual impact to *No More Food Fights!*

My office manager, Michelle Schrier, deserves appreciation for keeping my business moving along while I'm running around the world. You dealt with the wicked details of this book beautifully, which allowed me to think bigger.

Thank you to the clients across the United States and Canada who have entrusted me with "your people" for the last decade. You bring joy and meaning to my work, particularly when I see farmers reaching out and food buyers thinking differently as a result of our partnership.

I salute my professional speaker colleagues who helped inspire me to finally write this book, provide insight that the world outside of farming really doesn't understand haymows, and offer peer reviews. The same goes for the many advocates providing feedback and fodder.

Special appreciation to my closest girlfriends, who never know when their conversations with me will end up in a book or speech, but always support me. I treasure our friendship beyond words and am grateful for your perspective. I also respect your privacy enough to not share your real names with the world.

And last, but not least, thank you to my family who tolerates my driving passion for this work. My husband, who actually likes going to the grocery store, cares for our cattle and helps make it possible for me to do what I do. Our darling daughter, to whom this book is dedicated, is life's greatest blessing and a daily light in how important the cause of food and farming is to the future.

Table of Contents—Food Side

Introduction

A Journey Around the Grocery Store

"An empty stomach is not a good political adviser."

~ Albert Einstein

Going to the grocery store is one of my least favorite activities. I'm like many people who don't enjoy buying food anymore because it seems as though some special interest is trying to make me—and shoppers like you—feel guilty about nearly everything we put in our grocery carts or on our plates. Add in the confusion caused by conflicting ads and food propaganda on thousands of products. It's down right maddening!

Join me in a walk through a typical grocery store to see the forces at work in turning our dinner plates into a food fight. Greeting us on the right is the **deli,** filled with delicious sights and scents. I race past those foods, in fear that the fat and calories might attach themselves to my thighs or activate my sweet tooth.

Pretty **flowers** are on the left, but then I feel guilty about their carbon footprint, knowing the shipping and fertilizer it takes to bring those blooms. The roses probably came from the flower warehouse I visited in South Africa. But wait, aren't the flowers here because consumers wanted roses for twelve bucks?

The next case is what I call **specialty deli** items—15 different kinds of hummus, aged cheeses to pair with wine, mozzarella for caprese, ricotta for lasagna, pita chips, etc. This area makes me smile because it's the food we'll feed our friends when entertaining—and frankly, the labels aren't trying to sell me much more than enjoyment and indulgence. But specialty items are expensive!

Next up is the **produce** section, which you'd think would be another feel good place for a mom with a young child. But we live in the Midwest. Fruit and vegetables only grow here only a few months of the year, so there's no way we can always buy local. Being a "locavore" is fashionable, but will Midwesterners really settle for potatoes, turnips and a few apples all winter? Should we ban bread in Las Vegas?

Truth be told, about 45% of food in the US is imported—and this section of the grocery illustrates food miles. The food miles in produce are huge—mangos, bananas, grapes from another country; tomatoes, celery, peppers from the west side of the country; citrus from the southern states. Yikes! Thankfully I've seen the science that shows transporting in food is cheaper than trying to grow it in greenhouses in the dead of winter.

Staring at a carrot and thinking about its 35 billion genes makes me pause to consider science and the practical biotechnology that's resulted in seedless grapes and watermelons—to the delight of many kids and parents. Anything to make getting food on the table simpler!

Then I look at the **organic foods**, however, and wonder if I'm a terrible mom for not spending the extra dollars on that "luxury." I think of friends who grow products conventionally and organically and know both are a good choice—there's no need to feel guilty if you choose to not buy or simply can't afford organic. Besides, are the disadvantaged really better off only eating cheap fast food because they can't afford pricey organic. I don't think so! Do you?

Feeling annoyed, I'm thankful the **bread** aisle is next. My family loves bread—preferably homemade, but reality doesn't allow for that to happen too often so we buy bread. Whole grain, which is supposed to be the "right" thing to do, but then I remember hearing something about grain belly, growing tumors from the biotech products in that bread and poisoning our family with gluten.

So much for doing the "right" thing! Thankfully, a **dietitian** is in the aisle talking about the science showing the need for balance in a diet. I just know it's overwhelming to select from 75 varieties for a simple staple item and another 20 when we need bagels. Ugh! Is it time to go home yet?

Dried and **canned fruits** come up next. I always thought fruit was good and make sure our little girl has some at each meal to get those vitamins, but then the advent of high fructose corn syrup (HFCS)* "poisoning" made me ask if it's OK for us to eat anything but fresh food. Common sense and lifelong use of corn syrup in cooking reminds me that HFCS is simply a sugar, albeit one with a scary name.

Across the aisle is **peanut butter**—a favorite of the youngest member of our household. It's packed with protein, but what about all of the sugar and fat? And what do I know about the soil those peanuts were grown in? Then I recall the perspective from peanut farmers in the South as I asked questions about their soil care, as well as the nutritional studies about peanut butter being an excellent source of for brainpower at school.

The next couple of aisles are **sauces** and **baking items**. I snag some pasta and add to the carb load by grabbing a bag of flour and sugar. Then I get to the sandwich bags, where a wave of concern for landfills hits me before I turn to the **cereal aisle**. Staying away from the sugary cereals, I grab whole grain varieties and wonder how it's possible for farmers to get less than $0.20 of each box, as grocery prices rise and boxes get smaller. Is the farmer really the bad guy?

My mind again turns to biotechnology and how some people claim it's poisoning our food supply. This gets me a bit steamed since there's been extensive science supporting biotech. Then I think about others who believe that farmers in third-world countries are not allowed to use biotech seeds because of corporate control.

I know the truth is that dirty politics keep millions from receiving food donations that include biotech grain and it disgusts me. It's a tragedy that so many of those 'small holder' farmers cannot get the simple technologies that would radically improve their yields. In a fury, I leave the cereal aisle to turn to the **meat case**.

This is not a good choice, as I look at the **steak** that's claimed to be chock full of hormones, **pork** from pigs supposedly crammed in cages and **chicken** breasts laced with antibiotics. Then I remember that vegetables like broccoli and cabbage actually have more hormones in them than meat, the environments that pigs live

in are luxury resorts as compared the mud pits of yesteryear and science that shows humans use five times the level of antibiotics of those we use in animal agriculture.

As I reach into the **meat case**, I'm overwhelmed with disgust remembering sensationalized abuse videos that animal rights groups like to "release" to the nightly news. And even if animal rights messages don't make me feel guilty for being a carnivore, I think of Meatless Monday and how my hamburger is supposedly causing the planet to melt. I nearly knock over another shopper in my haste to get away from the meat case!

Thankfully, next is the **snack foods** aisle, where I'd gladly spend the entire shopping trip munching on crackers; however, our family knows moderation is key because we're the only ones responsible for our health and well-being. Besides, all the messages about the obesity make my hands shake when put snack food in my cart. Or maybe the shaking is because I know the **dairy case** is coming up, along with **eggs**, both of which are examples of labeling mayhem.

As I check my dozen of eggs for cracks, I notice phrases such as "cage free," "vegetarian fed," and "all natural." I'm confused because chickens are scavengers, which means they're eating manure in their cage-free, all-natural environment—if they survive predators. Gives new meaning to "you are what you eat!" Friends who raise **poultry** also assure me that chickens still prefer corn and soybeans, so that throws out vegan-fed as a special label. Besides, I know those birds' diets are more closely analyzed than mine, so I trust in the nutrition behind the eggs regardless of the system they're raised in.

Then it's time to look at **milk**, which used to be chosen based upon percentage of fat (skim, whole, etc.). Now dairy labels claim more things than my hairspray—antibiotic free, hormone free, no rBST, organic, grass fed and happy cows on marijuana.

The last is an exaggeration, but the others seem just as ridiculous to me as a dairy person because all USDA Grade A milk sold in grocery stores is antibiotic free and it all has hormones in it—and always has—since food comes from living things. All dairy milk has a lot of minerals and vitamins in it, making it a smarter choice rather than turning in the soda aisle in confusion. The rest of the label claims are more personal choice than anything.

My husband is a big fan of **Greek yogurt**, a newer product created in food science laboratories, so I throw some in my cart as I turn the corner, still shaking my head to clear the confusion from the label claims. At least the thought of new food creations give me a moment of bliss.

Happy thoughts of **ice cream** pull me into the frozen foods section. Our family tempers our love affair with ice cream with frozen yogurt, so I grab some after checking to be sure the sugar content isn't too high. While dreaming of ice cream for breakfast with smile, I happen upon **frozen vegetables** and am perplexed to see "all natural" on the generic store bag. What kind of vegetable isn't all natural? Isn't that common sense? 'Natural' is one of the most abused label claims. Get me out of here before I throw some veggies!

On the way to the cash register, I pick up a bottle of **water** and feel bad about plastic in landfills. But I need the water to wash down my Advil and bring some relief to the headache caused by going to the grocery store.

As I check out, I'm dumbfounded by the high cost of all this questionable food. I feel confused and guilty. Then I hear a person in the next aisle complaining about the food prices, with a finger firmly pointed at farm subsidies. "Nearly 80% of the "farm bill is for food assistance programs" was on the tip of my tongue, but I noticed the person behind me was ready to pay with a Supplemental Nutrition Assistance Program (SNAP) card—and I didn't want to make her feel bad. So I bit my tongue.

After throwing my groceries into the car in a temper, I spend the 20 minutes driving home through peaceful farm country trying to sooth my headache and sore tongue. **Why does food have to be so complicated?** All of those experiences at the grocery store mean I don't feel very good about what ends up on my family's food plates.

How about you? Friends tell me they find food confusing because all they really want is great tasting, affordable, healthy food for themselves and their families. **They would love to know where to get enough and information enough to feel good about their decisions.**

The politics and propaganda concerning the food on our plates is a frustrating problem for all of us. **Let's bring some peace to the plate.** My hope is that you can apply a couple of the six senses in this book on your next grocery store trip to help you make decisions about the food that is right for your family.

My Food Lens

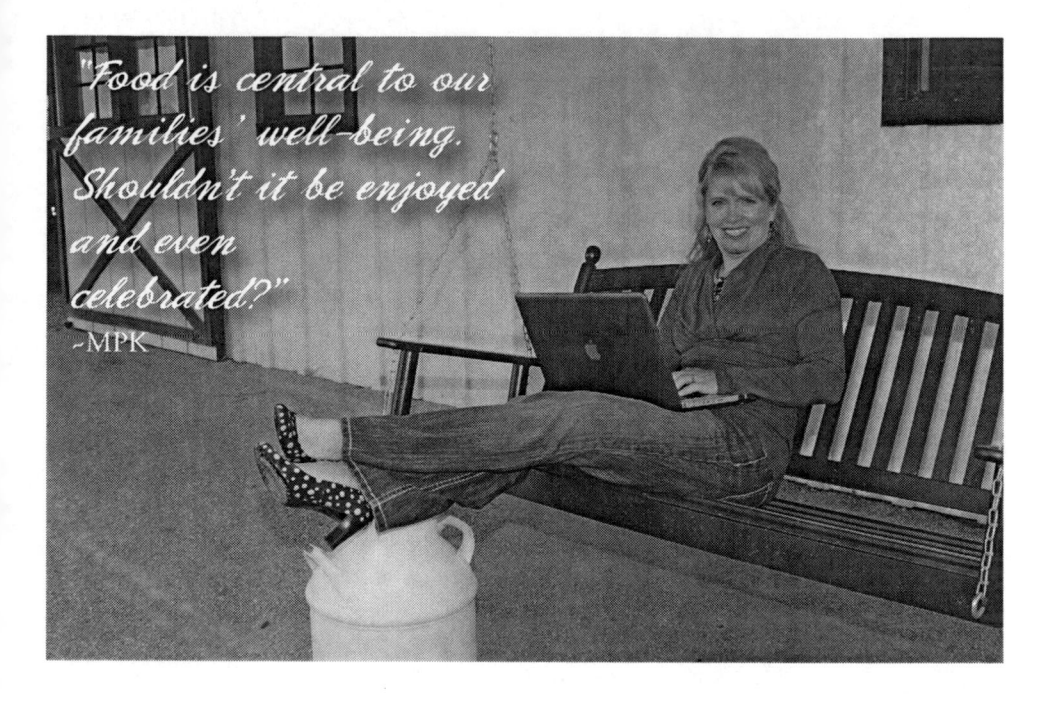

"*Food is central to our families' well-being. Shouldn't it be enjoyed and even celebrated?*"
-MPK

"**W**hat sense could you live without?" is a question I've never been able to answer. I'm extremely visual and experience the world through my eyes, and I love the sounds of friends, cattle, and music. I would wilt without the touch of loved ones. My nose can detect nasty odors about 10 times faster than most people (which is not an asset). And I'd likely weigh a whole lot less if I didn't find chocolate, wine, and crackers so very tasty.

So, it seems logical to me that all of the five senses should be our cues to a meaningful conversation, particularly with a subject like food. Food is a basic necessity; it does not have to be complicated or political. I don't believe there are rules that we all have to abide by. Food is full of personal choices.

A sixth sense is often overlooked—common sense. Sometimes when questioning yourself and the choices you're making for your family, it helps to stop and simply consider what makes sense. Common sense is defined as "good sense and sound judgment in practical matters." **Food should be good and be practical, right?**

What qualifies me to write this?

As we take a look at the six senses of food and farming conversations, I'll do my best to stay on the food side of the food plate. I've worked with food scientists, dietians, foodies, and chefs to gather their thoughts. I've baked bread since I was nine

years old, am known for my Italian dishes, and specialize in tasty low-fat creations (when there's enough time to cook).

You'll likely find that my farm roots and firsthand agricultural perspective sneak in, though—it's simply a part of my fabric (full transparency at **http://foodconvo. com/Qb8V0a**). This book isn't about spin or issue management as some naysayers will claim. It's deeply personal because of my farm perspective.

And when something is personal, it's tough to be objective or to extract emotions. That doesn't mean I think you are ignorant; I encourage you to balance my thoughts with your own perspective. Hopefully, we'll meet in the middle and it will leave us thinking. **Food is, after all, a personal choice.**

What qualifies me to write this book? I'm in the unique position of having a firsthand farm perspective and translating it to the non-farm public. I've been building communities to connect around the food plate in a variety of ways for 20 years. My love affair with food and farming started on a farm on southern Michigan, where I also learned to cook from a mother with a home economics degree. I've been breeding and judging dairy cattle as registered Holstein breeder for more than 30 years— and I'm thankful the view from my office still includes pretty black and white cattle on the small farm my husband and I built in west central Indiana.

Michigan State University provided my first glimpse of the marriage between farm and food as I went from dairy management to journalism to food science class while earning animal science and agriculture & natural resources communication degrees.

My career has led me from working with farmers in more than 25 countries, to managing corporate relationships across 15 states for the National FFA Foundation (a not-for-profit centered on agriculture education), to building a speaking business to help people connect the farm gate to food plate to fork. I am honored to have received the Certified Speaking Designation, awarded to less than 10% of professional speakers globally.

My work is very much a calling in both a professional and personal sense. I hope *No More Food Fights!* will make you think differently about food. I see a fork in the road between the farm gate and food plate—a divide that can be bridged through meaningful conversation. I don't believe that fork in the road has to be an 'either–or,' but should be a 'both.'

After all, food fights can be entertaining for a short time, but they get rather messy and smell bad when they've gone too far. Bystanders are hit with rotten tomatoes or fall down on the slimy floor. And the bullies who likely started the food fight slink away unnoticed, their pockets stuffed for another fight.

Is that really the scenario we want when we talk about food? I think not. Is all the negativity and grandstanding really necessary? Frankly, I'm tired of the food fight, the food rules and the drama around our food plate. **How about we try to grow the food conversation with civility, seeking connections around the plate?**

Why? Because it's the right thing to do. Because it's important to find some understanding—an intersection of values—in the debate around food. Because we

are personally involved with food at least three times per day. It sustains life. **Food is central to our families' well-being. Shouldn't it be enjoyed and even celebrated?**

I invite you to join me in adding decorum—a big word for common courtesy—to the debate. My hope is that you'll give serious consideration that the discussion around food and farming should include civility.

If all you can think of right now is "Yes, but... (they don't understand, I need to educate people, etc.)." I suggest you put the book down and reconsider your intent. Just know that you're smelling up the place for the rest of us and you'll eventually be throwing your rotten veggies at the mirror, so kindly take your fight to another room.

For the rest of you interested in exploring food with responsibility and respect, join me in the journey. **Let's move the conversation about food and farming to a different level.** You'll find the stories of people from all around the food plate shared throughout this book to make it a richer discussion with more diverse perspectives.

What you put in your mouth is a personal choice. What a farmer produces is also a personal choice. One should not overpower the other.

I hope this side of the book will help people most closely connected with food (grocery shoppers, dietitians, chefs, healthcare officials, foodies, retailers, et al.) find a framework for a more meaningful conversation with those in agriculture. *No More Food Fights!* is designed help you ask questions, explore the farm side of the plate, engage in a civil discussion, and arm yourself with a different way of thinking about food using six senses.

It is time to engage in a conversation about food that reaches across the plate so we can celebrate choice. You'll know which side of the book you need to read based on your role around the plate; those with food interests, start here. Those connected with the farm side, flip over. You'll find an identical chapter in the middle focused on connecting at the center of the plate.

Who knows? You might be interested enough to read the other side when you're done. Then I challenge you to share the book with a person on the other side of the plate. **My hope is that the ideas on each side will help grow a more meaningful conversation about farm and food.**

The Six Senses of a
Meaningful Food Conversation

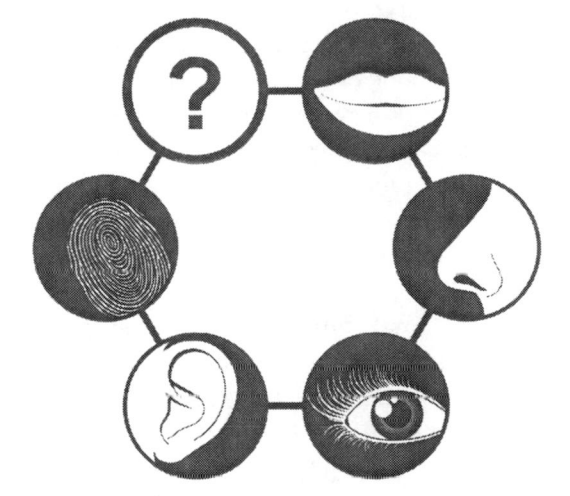

"There is no way in which to understand the world without first detecting it through the radar-net of our senses."

-Diane Ackerman

W hen my family sits down to a meal, the last thing we want to worry about is what kind of statement our food is making. **Food is about nourishment, and the meal is about spending time together as a family.** Yet the conversations outside of that table have become increasingly complex.

Talking about food didn't used to be like this; food was simply a basic necessity. Thirty years ago, going to the store was fairly straightforward. Certainly there were fewer options than the nearly 40,000 products[1] found in most grocery stores today, but food labels also weren't billboards for profit seekers. Food was just food, not a political statement.

Then we saw activist groups such as Greenpeace condemn technology used on farms, People for the Ethical Treatment of Animals (PETA) frame farmers as animal abusers through videos, Consumers Union trumpeting poorly researched claims about farm inputs, Farm Aid pitting small farmers against large farmers, and the smooth-talking Humane Society of the United States (HSUS) begin to attack modern farming practices. A decade ago, there were an estimated 25,000 anti-agriculture activists groups.

Then food retailers entered the game with propaganda campaigns in search of a niche to grow their margins. Labels began getting more confusing with claims about

the food inside of the package. Soon entire stores were built on the perception that one type of food was more superior to another.

Meanwhile, fewer people had any personal connection with where their food originated. Farms grew, adapted technology and changed practices out of necessity but did a poor job of talking to the public. The activist and marketing messages began to resonate with the majority of the population. The pendulum swung far enough that 1.5% of the population who farm and ranch was left with little influence in the discussion. Or so it feels.

Food isn't rocket science. It's grown on one end of the food chain and eaten on the other end. It's a basic necessity of life. And it certainly shouldn't be political. Yet, a disconnect began as the population shifted from rural areas to the city, not long after World War II. Now the chasm seems to be widening as agriculture modernizes and food interests heighten.

ROTTEN VEGETABLE 1
Approaching the conversation with stereotypes in mind limits your opportunities to have a robust conversation. Have an open mind as you learn about people around the plate and invite them to do the same.

If you're like the majority of people, you simply want to get the best food for your money. 95 percent of American consumers are classified as "food buyers"; people who choose foods based on taste, cost, and nutrition and who are neutral or supportive of modern agriculture practices.[2]

There's no need to be up in arms like those throwing rotten food around the discussions. Turn to your five senses and add a dose of common sense. **These six senses will help you make the choice that is healthy and ethical while meeting your social and environmental standards.**

The Food Marketing Institute reports Americans make an average of two trips per week to the supermarket. Rather than having those grocery trips be guilt-laden experiences, try this list of senses for your next walk through the grocery store.

1. **Touch:** reaching out to farmers
2. **Sight:** clarifying perspective
3. **Sound:** knowing what questions to ask
4. **Smell:** passing the science sniff test
5. **Taste:** feeling good about your personal choice
6. **Common sense:** remembering the basics

Keep at least two of these in mind on your next grocery store trip as you evaluate food, select from the menu at a restaurant or read a "nutrition" article.

I don't have all of the answers, but I do have a lot of questions. I also have strong convictions backed up by experience and evidence. However, I believe the conversation is bigger than one person, so I have woven personal stories of farmers, ranchers, food scientists, and dietitians into *No More Food Fights!*

Speaking the same language is a challenge around the food plate, so I tried to translate some of the crazy agricultural terms in a glossary that includes cow tipping, soil sampling and haymows—you'll find at the back of the book for terms marked with a *. Finally, there are links to many people and communities if you wish to reach across the food plate and connect on your own. The more people talking food in a civil way, the better.

My goal is to help you find guideposts for the conversation so you can reach across the plate, feel good about your food choices, and know where to turn for information when you want to grow the conversation.

We'll never agree on all the issues, but perhaps we can at least think about the people behind food a bit differently and find some commonalities. That would be far better than launching food grenades!

CHAPTER 1

Touch: How Can You Get in Touch with Farmers?

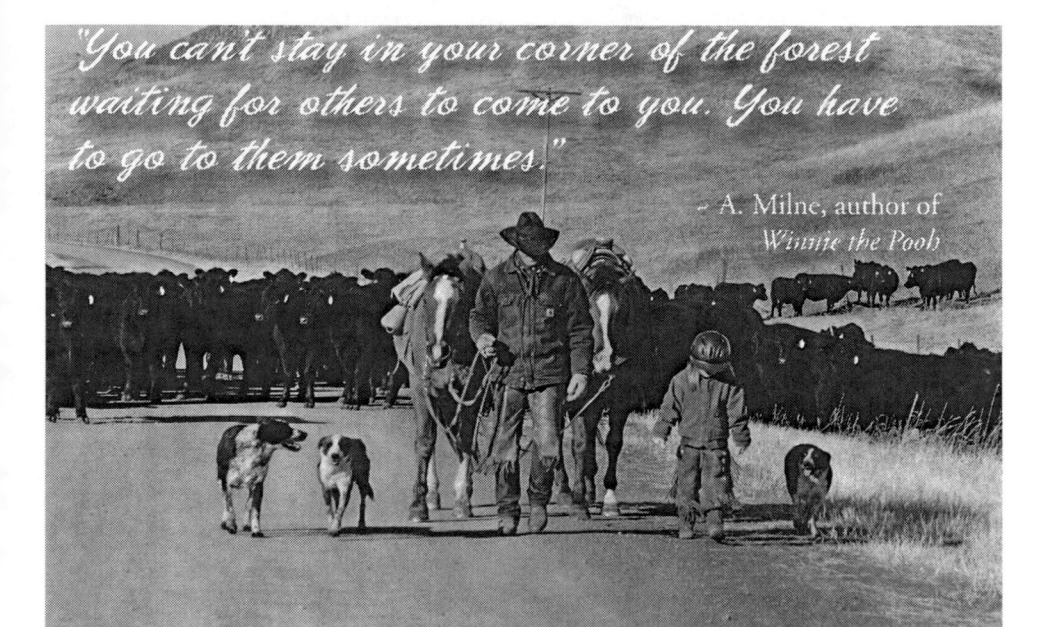

"You can't stay in your corner of the forest waiting for others to come to you. You have to go to them sometimes."

– A. Milne, author of *Winnie the Pooh*

"I just want to be able to find food that my family will eat that I can afford" was the response when I asked a close friend what she thinks about when she goes to the grocery store. As we talked over sandwiches at a local coffee shop on a sunny fall morning Justine added, "It's easier and cheaper to grab a frozen pizza than the fresh food I make that my kids probably won't like." We went on to commiserate how aggravating it is to see wrinkled noses after taking the time to make healthy food.

If you're like Justine, you don't spend a lot of time thinking about where that food came from, only how it impacts your family. I understand that, but I want to offer a perspective of why it might make sense for you to get in touch with farmers,

Farmers share many of your values, but aren't real great at talking about themselves. Let me share a bit of my personal story to illustrate some of the reasons why. My earliest memories go back to playing at the end of fields while my parents worked the land, chasing kittens in the haymow*, and feeding our dairy calves.

I thought this was a perfectly normal life, but I quickly discovered the opposite when I started school. My love of the farm was smiled upon as something "cute" when I was in elementary school and then questioned when I was in high school.

That baffled me, as I knew from a very early age that farming taught many life lessons.

Working with our veterinarian taught me science, biology, and anatomy. Picking stones (the not-so-enjoyable task of walking fields to get the rocks out of the way of equipment) taught me perseverance. Buying a $600 calf at age nine and a $7000 heifer at age 12 taught me more about entrepreneurship than any college course. Seeing my friends not really care where their food came from made me wonder why farming wasn't better understood.

What stereotype do you have of farmers? If you're like my schoolmates and professional speaking colleagues, you'll say I don't look like a farmer. Suffice it to say, I never really quite fit the farmer stereotype as a blue-eyed blonde. I like shopping, working out, wearing cute shoes, and enjoying the finer side of life as a foodie. I also enjoy working with animals ten times bigger than me and getting my hands in the dirt.

There are many others just like me in agriculture who don't fit the stereotypical farmer mold one bit. Amongst the thousands of farmers I've met, very few under the age of 70 wear overalls, just in case you're wondering.

Overcoming stereotypes

I'd like to introduce you to Amy, who originates from a city, has served in the Peace Corps, and just moved back to Wisconsin from Washington, DC. She wrote a piece at http://foodconvo.com/Tw0EhI about the stereotypes that can affect the conversation about food:

Stereotypes exist around the food plate that sometimes keep us from reaching out and finding true understanding.

Farmers wear overalls, drive pickup trucks, and are hardheaded. They go cow—tipping* on Saturday nights after the rodeo. They rarely travel outside the county line, and they definitely aren't using Twitter. Wrong.

City slickers wear shiny shoes, take taxis, and are arrogant. They couldn't tell the difference between a heifer* and a steer*, and they rarely get dirt underneath their fingernails. Wrong.

How can we help one another overcome these stereotypes to make real connections and find true understanding through our communication?

If you're more of a city person, then ask farmers about what they do and how they do it. They want you to know where your food comes from....

Waterbeds for cows?

Amy now sells waterbeds for cows, just to give you the rest of the story. Yes, farmers really do buy waterbeds for their cows to help them be more comfortable in their free stalls.* If you don't believe me, get in touch with her on Twitter and ask her why. You can find her at @AmyServes.

Hopefully, Amy's insight might give non-farmers a slightly different idea about people who work in agriculture. You may have gone to a farmer's market, visited a corn maze, or enjoyed a farm petting zoo. I encourage you to take a step further and

to employ the sense of touch by getting to know a variety of farmers for a more well-rounded perspective on the people behind your food.

It's easy to find farmers online blogging, tweeting, and facebooking. Many are sharing photos and snippets of daily life. Some even like to share videos from their tractors or barns (yes, they carry smart phones and know how to use them). If you want to visit farms in person, contact your state farm bureau to ask where you can find them, or take a look at the <u>Food & Nutrition</u> page on my website, where you'll find farmers from around the world.

The most important thing is that you identify your own concerns about food, rather than believing what's being told to you through the media, activists, or your friends. I will be the first to say there are bad apples out there who don't always do the right thing in caring for their farms, but the vast majority of farmers and ranchers are trying to do the right thing.

Do you judge all teachers and doctors because of a few bad apples? Likely not, so please don't use poor operators to form your only impression of farmers. After all, Amy will tell you there are farmers who put their cows on waterbeds.

FOOD CONNECTION POINT 1
Why ask why?

Asking questions of people at the right time can develop connections more effectively than a one-sided conversation. It uncovers the other person's needs or "hot buttons," which makes it a lot easier for you to connect with them. People will remember you because you showed interest in them.

Depending on your comfort level and the personality of the farm person you're talking to, there are many ways to ask questions. For example, you could try six basic questions: who, what, why, where, when, and how.

- How do you feel about the state of food and farming?
- Who really influences your business?
- What issues are important to you personally?
- Where are your customers?
- Why do you focus on _____?
- When is a crucial time of year for your business?

Why ask why? Because it is the best way to uncover hot buttons that help you develop personal relationships. Typically people with a sense of connection have a more civil conversation.

Beginning a civil conversation requires mutual respect and curiosity to get to know the other person. Farmers aren't opposed to talking with you, but reaching out to people different than them can be a stretch out of a farmer's comfort zone. You might feel the same way, but someone has to start the conversation and break the ice.

For example, I've needed to talk with farmers to learn about crops different than those grown on traditional Midwestern farms, such as peanuts. I did a little bit of research beforehand and then approached the conversation as an opportunity to learn. It was a bit awkward at first, but through asking gentle questions, I quickly found that the peanut farmers down south share similar values as I do. We chatted family and sports, with insight on how peanuts are grown in between.

As you approach the conversation with an agricultural person, it might help if you understand that modesty and independence run pretty strongly on the farm side of the plate. Look for common values such as family, technology, community, or sports. If nothing else, a farmer or rancher is always happy to talk (complain) about the weather!

How can we connect on commonalities?

It's hard to beat the feel of a new smart phone, the excitement in holding an iPad for the first time, or the delight in finding an app that makes your life easier. I love technology, especially since the day a PDA allowed me to carry my calendar in my palm.

Are you also an early adopter? I'd like to introduce you to my techno geek friend Darin. He worked on computers straight out of high school, gets his thrills out of analyzing data, and has a business helping others with precision technology.*

Darin is a very conservative Christian in northeastern Kansas. His wife is known for her baking prowess, which she's passing on to their three daughters. I can personally attest to their success in the kitchen. The couple's one son—the youngest of the clan—loves the iPad more than anyone in the family and "farms" in the basement year-round with his toy tractors.

The technology used in that family includes a GPS, two iPads, auto steer, a laptop, a Droid phone, two computers, remote radio controls for irrigation pumps, a yield monitor on the combine, moisture/temperature sensors in bin, GPS-assisted swath control, and precision controlled seed placement.* (check glossary for a translation) You see, Darin is a farmer. He farms a few thousand acres with his father. They have a family farm, passed along the generations, yet they likely use more technology in a day as you do.

He's concerned about protecting his soil and uses technology as a tool in that protection, while producing as much as possible. He's the first one to admit that he hasn't spent a whole lot of time thinking about what you want as a consumer. It's not that he doesn't care, but he's busy worrying about how to monitor the nutrients his soil receives, which genetics perform the best in various weather conditions, how to operate more efficiently, and what the market is telling the farm to do.

In spite of this, his care for the environment is a priority, as is running a business. And giving back to their small community is important, whether it's through providing jobs, purchasing supplies locally, or serving as a school board member. That is simply considered the right thing to do in their community, just as it has been for generations.

Although Darin's family may live and work in an environment very different from yours, he has many of the same values and priorities as you do and would likely love to geek out with other tech heads. You can reach him under the handle of @kansfarmer on Twitter.

As you get to know more farmers like Darin, you'll find they have values similar to your. I don't want to suggest you try to hug a farmer, but "reaching out and touching

someone" would go a long way in helping you understand where your food comes from. This can extend into the processing and retailing part of the food chain, as well.

Keep in mind, there is a lot of propaganda about farmers, but only 1.5% of the US population derives income from a farm or ranch. Rather than believing the stories, try getting in touch with a farmer—either in person or online—and gaining perspective on what it takes to farm today.

You'll likely find there's a wide array of farmers out there with diverse opinions on the right way to grow food. That's a good thing, because that creates diverse choices for your plate.

An example of a person who is seeking diversity on his plate and first-hand connection with farmers is former Olympic swimmer and now chef Garrett Weber-Gale. When I talked with him, he quickly listed questions he had for farmers.

> **FOOD CONNECTION POINT 2**
> Farmers aren't opposed to talking with you; they're just busy caring for their land and animals. Plus, modesty makes it difficult for them to talk about themselves. Look for commonalities you share to draw them out.

What are you growing? Why?
What did you grow 10, 20, 30 years ago?
Are you happy with where you sell?
Who controls your price?
How much depends on market, price, supply, and demand?
What do you need to continue progressing?
What questions do you have for me as a food buyer?

How about you? What questions and concerns do you have to ask farmers about?

Apples, corn and big farms—Oh my!

In interviewing people for *No More Food Fights!* an underlying concern about the shift that farms have made from a generation or two ago became clear. I asked a farmer friend in Michigan, Jeff VanderWerff, to provide perspective from his apple, corn, soybean, wheat, and peach farm on the shifts his farm has seen over four generations.

My family immigrated to the United States after World War I and started farming in 1947. Today, we raise corn, wheat, soybeans, apples, and peaches. Our story seems common in farming but is probably unique to many outside of agriculture. Over the last 20 years, agriculture in Michigan has become streamlined, vertically integrated, and very competitive due to the intense economic pressures our state has experienced.

We had what many would consider a typical farm when I was a kid. We raised a couple hundred acres of corn, wheat, soybeans, oats, and hay. We had about 30 cow—calf beef pairs and raised a few hundred hogs each year. It became more and more obvious that if we continued on this path in the late 1990s, it would be nothing more than a hobby, not a business. Our family couldn't make any money to live; we knew we had to specialize and

grow. By 1998, the cows, hogs, oats, and hay were all gone. We expanded our grain acreage rapidly, mostly from farmers who retired or were forced to sell out.

My brother and I were finishing college in 2004 and wanted to start to find our niche in the family farm. The answer, strangely enough, came in returning to what our family had given up: diversity. Joe and I started raising apples in 2005, then joined our dad and uncle as a single-family organization in 2010. Today, we have two distinct business units: fruit and grain.

Just as the crops are as different as night and day, so are many people's reactions when I tell them we grow grain and fruit. Somewhere along the line, traditional crop farming received a bad rap. Now, my family raises thousands of acres of corn and soybeans, and to us, the care of our land is very serious business.

We are obsessive about soil testing,* crop rotations,* and making sure we leave things better than we found them. The same is true for the apples; we don't like to spray dangerous pesticides.* In fact, we go out of our way to not use them whenever possible.

The perception seems to be that we are trying to do harm to the environment. Frankly, that is hurtful to me as a farmer. We care for the land; we have to, or we can't survive.

In my conversations with people outside of agriculture, I'm amazed by the reactions I receive depending on whether I tell them I raise fruit first or grain first. When the conversation starts with grain, first interaction is usually short: "Oh, you probably raise corn for ethanol." Yes, I do, and it's a major market for us right now; however, I have choices, and I can sell my crop anywhere. Right now, ethanol is the most profitable for me, so that's where it goes.

However, if I start out with saying I raise apples, I usually get tons of questions on how they are produced, where I sell them, etc. It seems that people are far more interested in learning about the food that they physically touch and where it originates. They are less interested in, and more easily swayed by propaganda, with products that are simply ingredients in food they buy, such as corn, soybeans, or wheat.

I'm glad to have the conversation and am constantly looking for ways to engage in conversation so that food buyers can see that we are in control of our own destiny, we know what we are doing, and we care—both about them and what we are doing.

Jeff falls in the extrovert category, rants about politics regularly on Facebook, and has a lot of dogs that he and his wife enjoy showing. Jeff started growing apples to diversify his family's farm, which made it possible for him to return home as a partner in the business. You can connect with Jeff on Twitter at @AgSalesman or look up his YouTube channel if you'd like to see how his family farms.

Hopefully, farmers like Darin and Jeff will help you be a bit more comfortable with the people behind larger progressive farms. I've been on farms across four continents and can tell you that there are great farms that are small, large, and every size in between.

If you're really concerned about what agriculture is doing with your food, try getting out of your corner of the woods and go see for yourself, whether in person or through social media. Tourist operations are great, but only going to that type of farm is kind of like experiencing only one kind of a coffee shop. Find large,

medium, and small operations you can get to know; compare them, talk to some more farmers, and then decide what food production system makes sense for yourself.

After all, you're the only one with the touch to know what is going to answer your food questions.

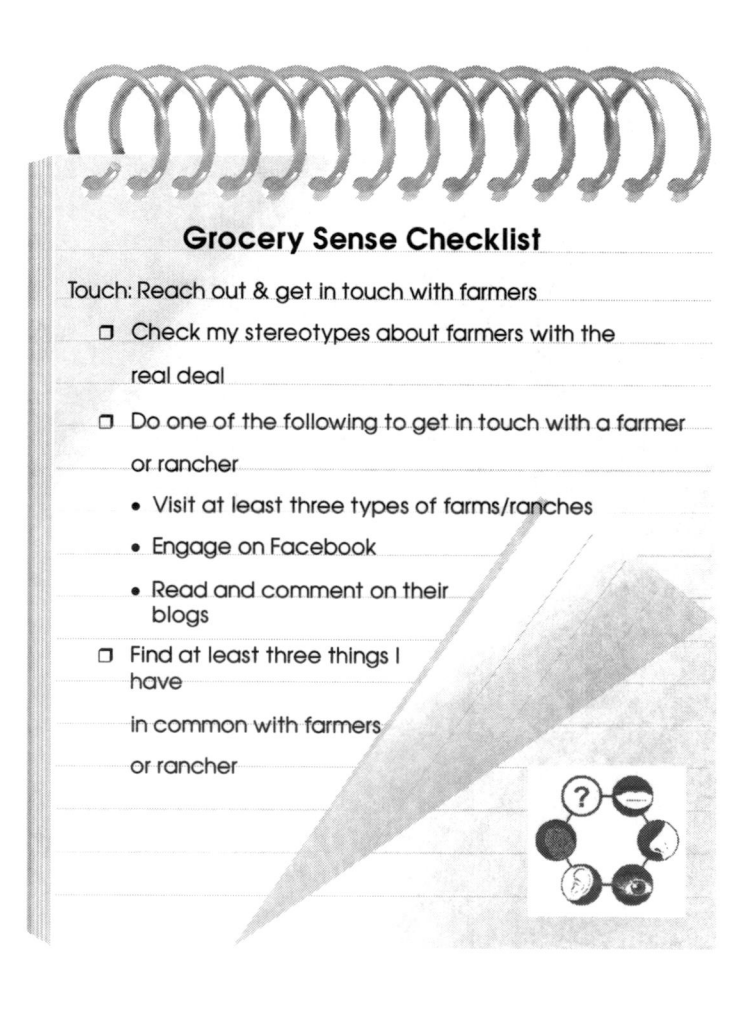

Grocery Sense Checklist

Touch: Reach out & get in touch with farmers

☐ Check my stereotypes about farmers with the real deal

☐ Do one of the following to get in touch with a farmer or rancher

- Visit at least three types of farms/ranches
- Engage on Facebook
- Read and comment on their blogs

☐ Find at least three things I have

in common with farmers

or rancher

Sight: How Can We Clarify Perspectives?

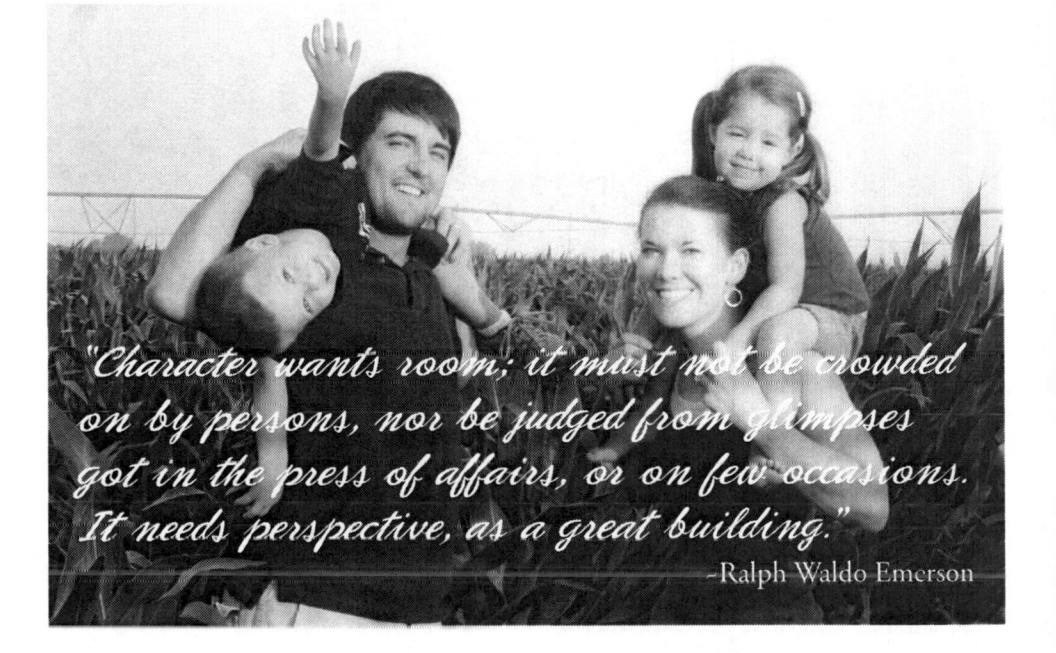

"Character wants room; it must not be crowded on by persons, nor be judged from glimpses got in the press of affairs, or on few occasions. It needs perspective, as a great building."

–Ralph Waldo Emerson

"He's having a hard time learning because he's hungry and probably didn't get enough sleep last night" a seasoned teacher gently told me one cold winter morning while I was volunteering at our local school." It immediately changed my perspective on the challenges teachers have to deal with in schools—and why some students struggle with learning.

Perspective can change the way you look at something in an instant. Working on a disaster-relief mission trip quickly clarifies for volunteers how deeply a natural disaster affects humanity. Learning that the person in front of you in line who is taking too long has a child stricken with cancer immediately softens your impatience with them.

It's no different with food; we gain perspective when we spend time with people on the other side of the plate. Agricultural people have a different food perspective because most of us grew up learning about caring for the land and animals. If you didn't grow up on a farm or ranch, your perspective may come from owning pets, being in

> **FOOD CONNECTION POINT 3**
> Food and farming are intensely personal choices. It's not our job to tell people that their choices are wrong. It's our job to speak from our side of the food plate and to reach across to understand the other side. How are you going to do that?

4-H, hunting, visiting your local farmer's market, or gardening.

That doesn't make us right and you wrong; different backgrounds mean our perspectives may be at odds, which can escalate the issues if we're not regularly talking.

Moms, kids and confined cows

A fellow professional speaker taught me the value of firsthand perspective and how city folk differ in their expectations around the food plate. She visited a modern farm, where she went from being skeptic of modern agriculture to finding moms just like her. Eliz Greene, a spokesperson for the American Heart Association, shared this perspective-changing experience at http://foodconvo.com/Tufp4G.

Ever wonder where your milk comes from? I got a chance to find out when I visited a dairy farm in Western Wisconsin and met 100 hard working dairy farming women.

Having only the media view of "factory" farming, I was firmly on the organic/free range/family farm side of the argument and a little concerned about visiting a large farm. I have to say my view has changed—still need more info, but it isn't as black and white as I thought. I visited a dairy farm with more than 800 cows—which is huge. It is run by a family (2 brothers and their wives) and some employees (total of 12 people I think). They'd like to have more help, but can't afford them with the low milk prices.

I had assumed "confined" cows would be unhappy cows, dirty cows, sad cows—but I was wrong. Over the hour-long tour, our host constantly talked about "cow comfort" from the different types of bedding to how the feed was presented. They invest in various types of fans and misters to keep them cool—they even had motion sensitive back scratching machines for the cows. It was a bit uncomfortable to watch one cow use it—she seemed to be REALLY enjoying it.

As anyone who has breast fed knows, if the mom is stressed or uncomfortable, the milk doesn't flow. I hadn't considered this concept in regard to dairy cows, but it makes sense. From that perspective, it seems ridiculous that a business person would set up a situation where conditions would limit production. No, indeed this farm was all about making the cows happy.

Our host talked about his routine and it was obvious how hard they work—long hours—and they are struggling to make a profit.

With their cute little kids running around it is hard to believe this was what an article in Time Magazine had called a "soulless" operation. Instead, I found moms I could relate to.

Anyway, here's what I've learned:

- *The farmers I met are VERY busy, care deeply, and deserve our respect.*
- *There's more to this issue than I ever imagined.*
- *I don't know enough yet—it is time to get more information and start really understanding where our food comes from.*

I suspect there is more than one right answer and the people who are most qualified to help me understand are the people working hard to produce our food.

It's amazing how visiting a farm can build understanding, isn't it? Eliz found moms like her, except their kids were in the barn. She could relate to the women through a shared perspective. **There's something about seeing with your own eyes and experiencing the conversation with people on the other side of the plate. It builds more than just understanding; it creates trust.**

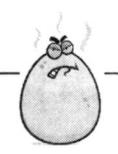

ROTTEN VEGETABLE 2
This is increasingly important in today's era of distrust. According to the book *How Risky Is It, Really?*, people are more afraid of business & industry, politicians, and processes that are closed and are less afraid (more likely to trust) consumer groups, neutral experts, and processes that are open.

Farmers who own larger farms have told me similar stories to Eliz's about visitors with preconceived notions. People will question where the part of the farm is that they abuse animals, what's being hidden from view, and why the farm doesn't look like what's been portrayed in the media.

Pardon me as I climb onto the farm soapbox for a moment. I understand it's nearly impossible to believe without seeing, which is why I started the six senses by stressing the importance of visiting farms.

If there's one thing I hope you'll remember from this book, it's that <u>farmers care</u>. We care about the land enough to use new technologies that reduce environmental impact. We care about our animals enough to see to their needs with respect and appreciation for the food they provide for humans. We care about our families enough to raise them on the farm in which we work. And yes, we care enough to build businesses around those interests and to add value to our communities.

Sustainability* isn't a trend or a catchphrase in agriculture; it's about being able to pass the farm on for generations. Farmers and the general public both value sustainability—and most all agree that sustainability has environmental, social, and economical components.

Recent research shows that 99% of farmers say they care about environmental practices and nearly 75% of consumers are concerned about the use of pesticides and insecticides in farming.[3] Now there's an opportunity for conversation!

But I digress. The point of this chapter on sight is to clarify perspectives. **Clarify your perspective with people who have firsthand expertise, whether that means a farmer, a dietitian, or a food processor.** Food can be so emotional, it is sometimes be hard to be rational when discussing it. Turning to those with firsthand expertise is a great way to gain a rational perspective.

I've had to do a perspective check, myself. When it was time to wean our daughter, I felt an immense amount of pressure to feed her right. After all, I had managed her health with my diet for her entire life and didn't want to mess it up.

Like a lot of new moms, I read *What to Expect When You're Expecting*, which listed the foods that are ideal for babies. My takeaway from it was that I would be a failure as a mom if her food wasn't 100% organic because farmers were pouring chemicals on our foods.

Funny thing was, I knew that farmers don't pour chemicals on crops—but I still was worried. I reached out to our pediatrician, a dietitian, and verified science (a sniff test covered in Chapter 4). It made me gain perspective that there are many ways to feed babies—just as there are many ways to parent children.

> **ROTTEN VEGETABLE 3**
> Expecting to find the worst when you visit a farm? There is not a special barn where animals are abused or poisons hidden. Even if you're concerned farmers don't put animal care first, farmers are far too straight forward and worried about efficiency to be pulling such antics.

Sometimes clarifying perspective is just a matter of checking information out for yourself to have a sense of trust that you are doing the right thing. Find one food that's bothering you and invest a week in finding perspectives from around the food plate. You might be surprised at how much more trust you have.

London bridge is falling and so is farming

A civil conversation might be easier if we simply think about food as a bridge. Literally. I thought Jennifer Heim, a structural engineer, made a lot of sense when she questioned whether the public trusted engineers more than farmers:

Recent studies have shown that consumers trust farmers, but not farming.[4] As a structural engineer almost no one I know (including my farmer husband) actually understands what I do. However, I also don't know anyone who hesitates before walking into a building or driving over a bridge.

So the question is—why? Why do people question the way that farmers grow their food but not the way the engineers design their buildings or other infrastructure? I first thought the difference in reactions must come down to differences between farming and engineering. My roles at my office and at our farm are extremely different...aren't they? Thinking about the occupations at a basic level (beyond tasks), I only came up with three differences.

Educational requirements

When I first meet someone new and mention that I'm a structural engineer, their reaction is usually a blank stare followed by "is that like an architect", but occasionally it's "wow, you must be smart". When I tell a new acquaintance that my husband is a dairy farmer, the reaction is somewhat different.

Most don't seem to know what to say, maybe because they aren't familiar or comfortable with farming. But of all the varied responses I've gotten, not once has someone said, "Wow, he must be smart." For the record, he is smart (and has a degree), but farmers aren't required to go to college and engineers are.

Emotional connection

Not many people have an emotional connection with steel or concrete. Engineers design structures made of these faceless, lifeless materials with faceless lifeless calculators and computers. Animals and plants are a different story. Farmers work with living things,

things people worry about. How do you feel when you see a baby calf or a healthy garden? What about a concrete slab or steel beam? Even as an engineer, my emotional connection is quite different.

Media influence

Part of the public's reaction to anything is related to what they hear from the media. How has the media portrayed engineering? They haven't. If I recall the results of the 2007 Minneapolis bridge collapse investigation correctly, the bridge failed because of an undersized connection—an engineer made a mistake.

I only know that because I read part of the report. On local news I recall hearing about some high percentage of bridges in Missouri that had failed inspections and were still open, placing the blame on government. It wasn't true, but I never heard that from the media. Conversely, the media has certainly addressed modern farming—and usually not in a positive light. Unfortunately, that's all many people hear or see.

Jennifer Heim is a structural engineer working in Kansas City and blogs at http://heimdairy.wordpress.com. She has both B.S. and M.S. degrees in Civil Engineering from the University of Illinois. In her free time, she helps her husband David operate their small conventional dairy in northeast Kansas. See the complete post at http://foodconvo.com/QITmg2.

Although it might seem a bit odd to think about food as cement, it might help us to remove some of the emotion from the conversation and avoid the "London bridge is falling " mentality. Perhaps it would allow us to find more common values, regardless of our positions on the food issues.

How many hands are on your food?

Pursuing degrees simultaneously in animal science and in agriculture & natural resources communications at Michigan State University put me in quite a breadth of classes (not to mention how it occupied both sides of my brain). One of my favorite parts of my education was the diversity of classes that provided a panoramic view of our agrifood system: Food Systems Management on the many steps between gate and plate, Packaging on how a package can change products, and Food Science on the complexities of creating food.

That background likely set the stage for my appreciation of different parts of the food chain. Today's agrifood system is both an asset and a curse; it is a case study of efficiency and progress—but if one part fails, it creates questions about the whole.

Processing of food seems to bring up concern in food circles, but I'd suggest a different look at it. I could point to studies that show frozen vegetables can be healthier or that you likely wouldn't enjoy an unprocessed chicken running around your kitchen, but I'll refrain. Washing a vegetable is processing it. Creating products that are kitchen staples such as corn starch, baking soda, and salt require processing.

I've sat at the table with people with PhDs in food microbiology and found them just as confused as I am about the hysteria in the food conversation. They don't understand why science in food is a bad thing; they spend their days researching food to determine ways to make food better. It's frustrating to be misunderstood, regardless of your position around the plate—food buyer, farmer, or microbiologist.

Here's a more scientific look at the roles around the plate from John Copland, PhD and professor of food science at Penn State. He brings an interesting perspective to the importance of others—beyond the farmer—in the agrifood system.

Farmers are essential in our food system. Without farmers we would all starve, but farmers don't make food. There is almost nothing produced on farms that is immediately edible. Post-farm processing can be so minor you scarcely notice—wash the apples, it can be significant but traditional—mill and separate wheat to make bread flour, or it can render the source material unrecognizable—separate the corn starch then digest with enzymes to make high fructose corn syrup.

All of these are food processing and are required to turn farm produce into food that people eat. So what are the connections between the farm and the table? There are many possibilities, but let's start by following the path taken by most of our food.

Almost all food processing in the developed world is done at an industrial scale. The supermarkets and restaurants we buy most of our food from in turn buy their supplies directly or indirectly from other companies that make it. These companies in turn buy their ingredients from other companies and so on until someone pays the farmer for the produce to feed the cycle.

A simple example is tomato ketchup—tomatoes, salt, vinegar, and spices. The tomatoes were grown by a farmer, ground and concentrated into paste in one factory, then shipped to a second factory to be blended with salt, vinegar, and spices, cooked, and bottled as ketchup. Sure, without farmers, the food system wouldn't happen, but the same could be said for the retort operators, truckers, microbiologists, sensory scientists, and factory workers.

It's difficult to explain the complexity within the constraints of this chapter, as the modern agriculture system is worthy of its own book. Suffice it to say that even the simplest food has likely had a tremendous number of hands on it—in a good way.

Let's take a look at an apple. A scientist was involved in developing the right variety of tree, an agronomist worked on selecting the inputs to be sure the apple doesn't have worms, the farmer oversaw the production, a microbiologist researched how the apple plays with other foods, a trucker hauled it from the farm to a packaging site, a processor washed and packaged the apple, a grocer made it available to you, and then you drove it home. The process may seem scary to some, but a simple apple has a story of people and science behind it that protects you while meeting nutritional needs.

Counting on experts in animal welfare

Now to turn to the animal side of the business, which gets to those emotions that my engineer friend Jennifer mentioned earlier. Like many pet lovers, I find it hard to resist a fuzzy little kitten or puppy dog playing. My childhood memories center around animals—trying to persuade the Saint Bernard to pull me on a sled, raising orphan kittens rescued from the barn, and having calves as playmates.

I also recall going to local animal shelters as a child and feeling terrible for the animals who had no home, so I understand the attraction to campaigns run by the

Humane Society of the United States (HSUS). After all, who wants to see these cute little creatures suffer?

The reality is that HSUS advertises to attract animal lovers' dollars. Many great people and organizations have contributed because they want to help animals. An *Animal People News* article has shown that HSUS contributes more to its $11 million pension plan than to local shelters.

Why? Take a look at "The Myth of the Humane Society of the United States," a law school article that outlines how the bulk of the HSUS's income was spent on fundraising, campaigns, and lawsuits:[5] "There is one minor detail left out of these commercials. The Humane Society of the United States is not a large network of animal shelters, as it would have you to believe. In fact, the HSUS does not own, operate, or lease a single animal shelter in our country."

Contrast this type of political activity to that of people who work with animals every day. It's similar to the debate around government and education. Do you trust the people who are working with students daily to deliver education the most effectively—or those who are creating a system? As a mom, I trust teachers trained in education and deal with the challenges students bring to school with them, and I expect them to make the best decisions related to education. While I understand the importance of national and state standards, I also see such standards limiting the true experts—teachers—and I value the firsthand expertise of those teachers far more than I trust government in setting educational standards.

When it comes to farm animals, firsthand expertise means a farmer knows when an animal isn't feeling right by looking in the animal's eye. The farmer knows how to best handle the situation based on experience, data about the animal, and the farmer's ongoing education. Farmers work with state and national organizations to adhere to best practices as standards. Just as a reference point, the larger the farm, the greater the standards.

It troubles me that some studies show activist organization such as the HSUS as one of the expert sources in animal care. Farmers are deeply committed to the animals in our care and consider it a privilege to care for those animals so they can provide food. If an animal is in distress, farmers will spring into action to help. Please keep this in mind next time someone shows a new "shocking video" about the treatment of animals on farms. **Go to a farm and see with your own eyes—or clarify your perspective with a true animal-care expert, such as a veterinarian.**

For example, an illustration of the importance of proper animal care on a farm, both for animal welfare and business profitability, is provided by Dr. Kathy Swift. Kathy is a wine-loving artist who also happens to be a veterinarian and a mom of three young boys. If you think farmers are driven more by profit than by caring about the well-being of their animals, you might want to consider the scientific evidence that clearly shows that a farm's profit suffers if its animals are routinely mistreated because the animals won't grow.

Happy cows isn't just an advertising slogan; it's something farmers strive to make happen every day. Growing up on a dairy farm, I still remember that even at a young age, treating animals with kindness and respect was important to the farm's success. It wasn't

until years later that I actually learned the science behind the importance of a neighboring farm's mantra, clearly displayed in their barn, "Speak to the cow as if she were a lady."

It comes down to the stress hormone, cortisol. Cortisol (known as hydrocortisone when taken as a prescribed anti-inflammatory medication) is activated whenever an animal is under stress. This hormone is very important in that it plays a big part in the "fight or flight" phenomenon. Its release causes a chain reaction that causes the body to raise blood pressure, accelerate the action of the heart and lungs, and dilation of blood vessels going to the muscles.

All of these are important in the animal's ability to protect itself and escape a dangerous situation. We know, however, that animals exposed to stress for extended periods of time experience chronic cortisol exposures.[6]

The constant release of cortisol is counterproductive to many things, including milk production, fertility, and muscle growth, just to name a few. Side effects from cortisol release may be temporary stresses, such as being sick from disease or being moved to a new group of animals, or may be from a longer term stress, such as poor feed quality or inadequate housing to protect the animals from the weather elements.

So what do farmers do in order to minimize the stress animals experience on their farms? These are considered best practices.

- Move and work with the animals without using loud voices and noises, stick, electric prods and anything else the animals may find bothersome.
- Provide an environment where they can be clean and comfortable, have access to fresh, quality feed and water, and where they can interact with their herd mates in a safe manner.
- Treat illnesses in a prompt fashion, including providing for an animal's pain alleviation needs.

I am excited about where the future of animal welfare is going. Not only do we realize alleviating pain is important, but research is expanding in this area. Future medicines will give us more options to effectively manage the pain and discomfort of food producing animals.

There is also the use of technology involving animal behavior—everything from recording the number of steps animals take in a day to monitor their daily well-being to using thermal imaging to non invasively determine their health status. These will be invaluable for farmers, helping them produce safe food in the best way possible.

Animal care isn't an afterthought in what we do in agriculture; it's at the forefront of what we do every day. I see farmers on a daily basis that care deeply about their animal care, whether they have a large farm or small farm. It's certainly my top priority as a veterinarian. Just because an animal will end its life as a source of food doesn't mean that it shouldn't be treated humanely while it is alive.

Dr. Swift holds herself—and the farmers she works with—accountable to these standards. If you have questions or want to be amused by her combination of art, manure, wine, and animal tweets, connect with her at @CowArtandMore on Twitter.

Perspective check is an important part of a meaningful conversation. Social media has developed many incredible connections and communities for people with

food interests, such as FoodChat on Twitter or Foodthanks (http://foodthanks.com) that happens the day before Thanksgiving. Unfortunately, social media has also provided a bully pulpit for those with one-sided agendas.

I'm thankful that the majority of people simply have questions about their food. My hope is that your sense of sight is simply a reminder to get a fuller perspective on food and farming claims from experts—those with firsthand experience. Again, pick one issue you're concerned with and spend a week doing a perspective check.

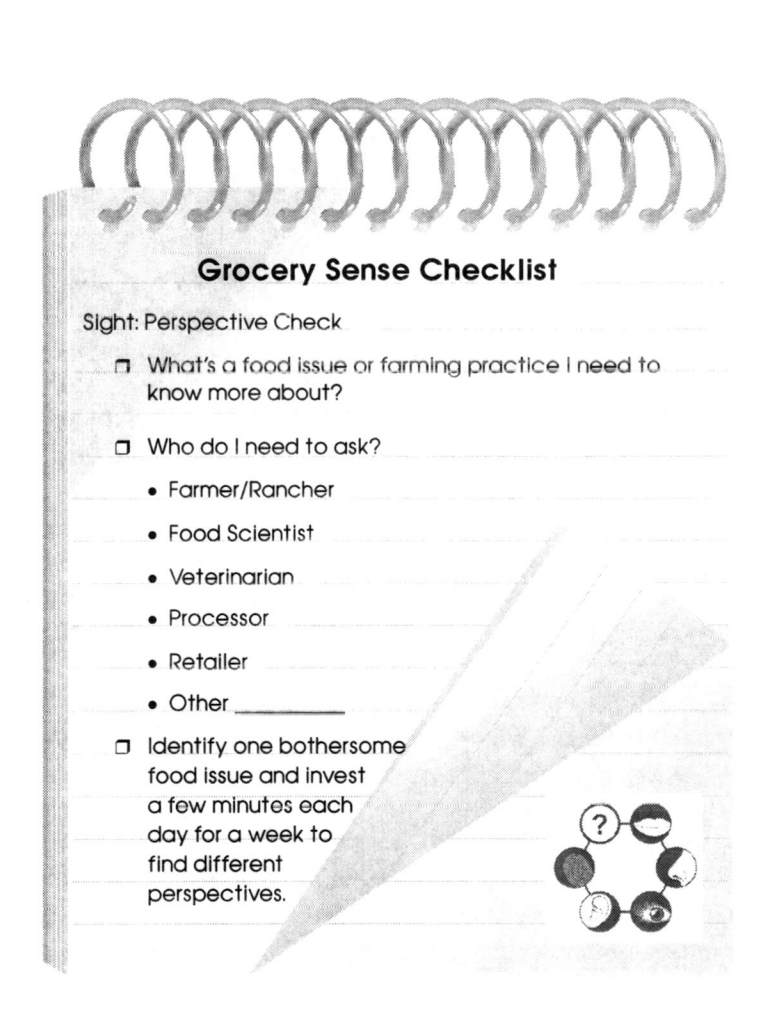

Grocery Sense Checklist

Sight: Perspective Check

☐ What's a food issue or farming practice I need to know more about?

☐ Who do I need to ask?

- Farmer/Rancher
- Food Scientist
- Veterinarian
- Processor
- Retailer
- Other _____

☐ Identify one bothersome food issue and invest a few minutes each day for a week to find different perspectives.

CHAPTER 3

Sound: Do You Know What Questions to Ask and How to Listen?

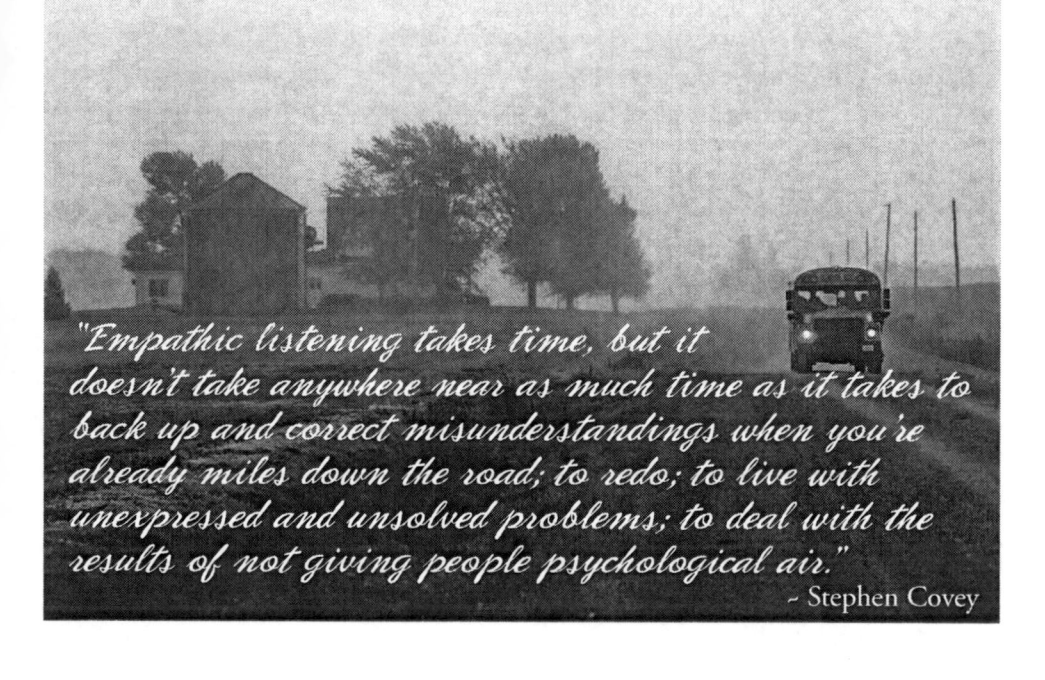

"Empathic listening takes time, but it doesn't take anywhere near as much time as it takes to back up and correct misunderstandings when you're already miles down the road; to redo; to live with unexpressed and unsolved problems; to deal with the results of not giving people psychological air."

~ Stephen Covey

The best tools for having a conversation are attached to your head and will also help you make a decision about your food. Fortunately, you have two ears and only one tongue, though many act as if that ratio is reversed. I highly recommend biting your tongue when others are talking, particularly if you're trying to develop an authentic connection.

Questions as a key ingredient in healthy conversations

One of the best ways to develop an authentic connection to ask really good questions—questions that will make the other person think a bit and provide you with perspective, as we discussed in the last chapter.

Eliz, my speaker friend who shared her perspective changing farm visit in Chapter 1, lists questions that she, as a healthcare professional, would like to know from farmers:

- What should I know that I don't?
- What do I think I know that is just plain wrong?

- What should I be reading?
- Who should I rely on for good, unbiased, information?

When I did a quick poll on Facebook asking ag folks what they really wish you'd ask of them brought a slew of questions. They suggest folks on the other side of the plate ask farmers and ranchers:

- Why do you do what you do?
- Do you think the food you grow is safe?
- Where does the food go when it leaves your farm?
- What kind of farm subsidies do you get?
- What percentage of the food dollar do you get, and why?
- How long does it take to get food from gate to plate?
- Are you controlled by agribusiness?
- Why do you use biotechnology? Isn't the food from it dangerous and unhealthy?
- Do you farm differently from your grandparents? Why?
- Do you give your animals antibiotics? Why? Do the antibiotics end up in the meat/milk?
- You use chemicals on your crops. Isn't that poisoning all of us?
- Do you have a lot of money? You certainly have a big house and buildings.
- Do you feed what you raise to your own family?
- What do you wish would be different in agriculture?
- Show me how you farm and raise animals. Is what I see and hear the truth?

The agrifood system is a complex business with many layers complicated by an increasingly international marketplace. It certainly isn't perfect, but it has been built around market demands. And those demands have certainly changed over the past few decades, as evidenced by the food made available to us in the grocery store.

Let's take a look in my kitchen as an example. Fresh ingredients are my cooking preference, but that is balanced by price and time. I'm thankful for the jar of pasta sauce I can pull from my pantry, even if it includes tomatoes from California, mushrooms from Canada, and herbs from the upper Midwest all coming together at a processing plant on the East Coast. It meets the USDA standards, is economical, and makes meal prep a lot faster.

My family also enjoys the pasta sauce we made this summer with tomatoes, eggplant, peppers, and herbs from our own garden, but it took about 10 hours longer to make—and that's just not always practical for two working parents. Thus, the multilevel system between farm and your food plate. It's been developed out of necessity—and market demand. **Cooking—and eating— doesn't have to be an either—or situation. You decide what's right for you.**

Charlotte's Web, agribusiness or farmer?

Given the hours we spend raising vegetables before they're even simmering into a sauce, I'm always amazed by the beautiful produce we find in the store. Shay Myers, along with his family in Oregon, is one of the farmers who makes that happen at Owyhee Produce. His family's products go to retailers, processors, and wholesalers. He and his family have grown barley, beans, corn, mint, onions, peas, shallots, sugar beets, and wheat for generations and recently added asparagus, chipollinis, and shallots for the fresh market. Shay has some interesting experiences with his "farmer" label.

When I was in my teens, I thought I had the best life there was. It wasn't until I moved to Los Angeles at the age of 20 that I realized how "un-cool" being a farmer was. I would tell people I was a farmer and they would just kind of look at me and smile, as if I didn't have a clue.

It wasn't until I started asking people who reacted that way, WHY was that their reaction? The usual response—"so you have a few cows, chickens, and a red barn, that is... great."

You see, for them, food came from the grocery store. What I did was perceived as more of a hobby than a way to feed people. Because of that, I wasn't sure if I was going to be a farmer during college. And I sure wasn't going to tell people that's what I wanted to be.

Then after college, when I had decided to come back to the farm, I started calling myself an agri-entrepreneur so people wouldn't look down on what I did for a living as much. It has taken me a long time to get here, but the fact is what I do for a living is actually pretty cool. I am not sure that "farmer" really alludes to the reality of what I do for a living to an urban dweller, but it suits me.

Farmer suits me because the other name I could call myself is "agri-businessman." The same Angeleno (that's what we call folks from L.A.) who looked at me blankly when I called myself a farmer looked at me a destroyer of Mother Nature. The word "agribusiness" just had a negative feel to it—my tractors may as well have been the machines in Dr. Seuss's Lora that destroyed entire trees just to make a single toothpick. So you see, being called a farmer may have its downfalls, but so do the alternatives.

Today I run a business, along with other members of my family, which does $10 million in gross annual sales. We employ nearly 60 full-time employees, and we farm over 3,700 acres. We also drip irrigate a large percentage of our crops, saving 30% of Mother Nature's water. We rotate our eight distinct crops on a five-to-seven year rotation; this builds humus* and reduces erosion.* Our tractors have been updated to tier 4 engines, reducing fuel consumption by 25%.

We truly believe in commonsense farming practices—practices that ensure not only safe food but also allow a farmer to be profitable and ensure long-term existence. We all have different ideas and philosophies about life and earning a living. Just like in the city, farms differ in that regard.

Organic farming is good and will support a single family, but a large multigenerational farm like ours could never make it. We have to look at things on a larger scale. Large-scale farming creates efficiencies that can't exist on small-scale farms. It also allows for Good Agricultural Practices (GAP) and food safety standards that are impossible otherwise.

We invest in technology that allows us fewer trips through the field and increases yield. This product also prevents produce from rotting on the shelf or in your pantry. Some would respond to this and say that any artificial manipulation of Mother Nature is wrong and we should not "play with our food." I always have to ask if that same person will take medication to get rid of a headache, lower their cholesterol, or prevent pregnancy.

So what is the difference? Perception and culture. Too many perceive farming and its culture as an idealistic existence, one that doesn't require much thought but instead requires only work. At the same time, a farmer's culture prevents her from intervening to change the negative perceptions.

As a farmer, I am constantly battling an invincible foe, Mother Nature. She can destroy a crop and an entire year's earning in a single hailstorm, so when I am criticized for using chemicals, hybrid seeds, and artificial fertilizers, my attitude is one of passivity. As a farmer, I fight the battle I think can win or I wait out my foe, as we're accustomed to doing with Mother Nature. This is the wrong attitude when it comes to culture and perception, but it is still the case.

So as a farmer, I have to run a business while trying to change both my own cultural inculcation and that of society as whole. As a part of that, I am happy to answer questions.

You can find Owyhee Produce in Oregon, on Facebook, or at www.owyheeproduce.com. It's a great chance for you to connect with a produce grower and to learn more about their practices (this is even something that most traditional farmers could benefit from, but don't tell them I said so).

If you're like me, Shay's comments stimulated all sorts of questions for you and his story is a wake up call that *Charlotte's Web* doesn't represent today's farms. **What questions do you have about how your food is grown and gets to your plate? Who do you need to ask in the food system?** Write them down at the end of this chapter, or if you're reading this digitally, grab a piece of paper and jot down your questions.

Processors, politics and perspective check

As you think about the questions you have about food and who you need to ask, you may realize that your questions are broader than those the farmer can answer. It might be a processor or retailer. To help with that perspective, I'd like to introduce you to my friend Amy, a small processor in southern Kentucky, who will be the first one to tell you that farmers don't make food.

A fiery short little southern woman, Amy is a mom of three who does the work of a few men with her husband at their small processing plant, John's Custom Meats, a modern on-farm USDA slaughterhouse, processing facility, and retail meat market. Among performing a laundry list of other duties, Amy navigates the Food Safety Inspection Service (FSIS) regulatory world, serves as the in-plant food safety coordinator, and consults with livestock farmers on ways of adding value to their livestock. She's an example of a processor who turns raw product from the farm into a consumable product. She had this to say at http://foodconvo.com/SoNnZ6:

We are in a unique position. Politics and regulation pull us in one direction; consumers are pulling us in another, and livestock farmers? They pull us every way but loose! We generally are stuck in the middle. Regulations dictate the feasibility of what slaughter & processing services my business offers and how I go about offering them (for the most part). Consumer concerns and requests shape our wholesale and retail meat product offerings. Our livestock farmers are so diverse their needs are all over the place.

On the processing side of the business, we provide services for a diverse range of livestock farmers. They are conventional to organic, internationally owned to family owned, large commercial to the small family homesteader, dairy operations and cattle, pigs, lamb, goat, and exotics. My customer base is an eclectic mishmash of agriculture sectors, related but unique with their own individual needs.

Whether their customers are their own family, the general public, or the commercial commodity market, they all have at least one thing in common. Me. They need me and I need them. Neither of us could successfully exist without the other. Our retail & wholesale clientele are equally diverse. This perspective has given me an appreciation for farmers and consumers of all walks of life. They all (for the most part) come together to meet in the middle in the most unlikely place…at the processor. Who knew? Developing an understanding and tolerance is essential to our success. Not just my businesses success, but agriculture as a whole.

Farmers often feel like they are under attack, and many times rightfully so. Consumers may feel as if no one is listening to their concerns, usually equally warranted. Many times, we as farmers get caught up in "fighting back" with science jargon we likely don't fully understand ourselves and preaching industry factoids instead of hearing, acknowledging, and connecting on a human level.

We're often found bickering amongst ourselves like school age children instead [of] sharing our experiences in meaningful debate. This is no surprise because benefit to one sector of agriculture may well likely result in injury to another. I think we can do better at understanding and respecting each other.

By the same token, some outside of agriculture make narrow minded demands on already struggling farmers to make the world of agriculture a fictional fairyland. Agriculture is not black and white. It is all shades in between, thankfully. "Factory Farm" is an offensive, dirty word— and sure to put a farmer on the defensive.

Conventional farming is not trying to kill you. Organic farming is not a cure all. Local food economies cannot feed the masses, they won't cure world hunger, nor will they save the world from certain demise. However, all of those types of farming combined

together is a thriving agricultural community with diverse product choices to meet the needs and wants of many.

If you're on Twitter, follow Amy at @kyfarmersmatters for an entertaining stream, all things meat, and an education about bourbon.

Although thoughts of it don't create bucolic images, the agrifood system is a multi-tiered system that fails if one component doesn't work with others as food goes from farm to fork. The next time you read a report about how food is going to make you grow three heads and walk like a frog, I'd suggest you think about some of the people in *No More Food*

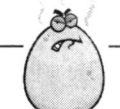

ROTTEN VEGETABLE 5
These are romantic visions of what a farm should look like. Just as hospitals and schools have been updated with technology, modern farms don't necessarily fit Charlotte's Web imagery. Some farms still have pretty wooden barns; others operate with metal grain bins larger than the house. Neither is wrong; they're just different. Wondering why facilities have changed? Common sense might point to people taking better care of the land or animals. Just ask if you're concerned.

Fights! and ask yourself these three questions:

- What does the original study cited by the media actually say?
- Are there multiple sources cited with firsthand experience?
- Does the claim make ethical, business, and common sense?

To summarize what I have been saying about the sense of sound: **use your head to ask questions of the people with firsthand experience in agriculture and food.** Even more importantly, **use your ears to listen even when you don't agree with what you're hearing.** If it makes you feel any better, I asked the ag folks to leave scars in their tongues while listening to your concerns.

As Steven Covey notes, empathic listening could go a *long* way in clearing up misperceptions around the food plate. How 'bout you try it out?

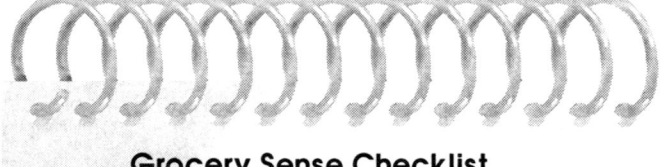

Grocery Sense Checklist

Sound: Questions & Ears

☐ Commit to empathic listening for the next 24 hours, regardless of the conversation.

☐ Engage someone from another part of the food plate in a conversation.

Who am I asking?

_____

_____

_____

What's my question?

_____

_____

_____

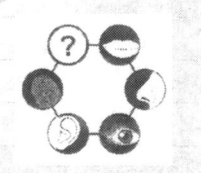

Smell: Does it Pass the Sniff Test of Science, Sensationalism or Celebrity?

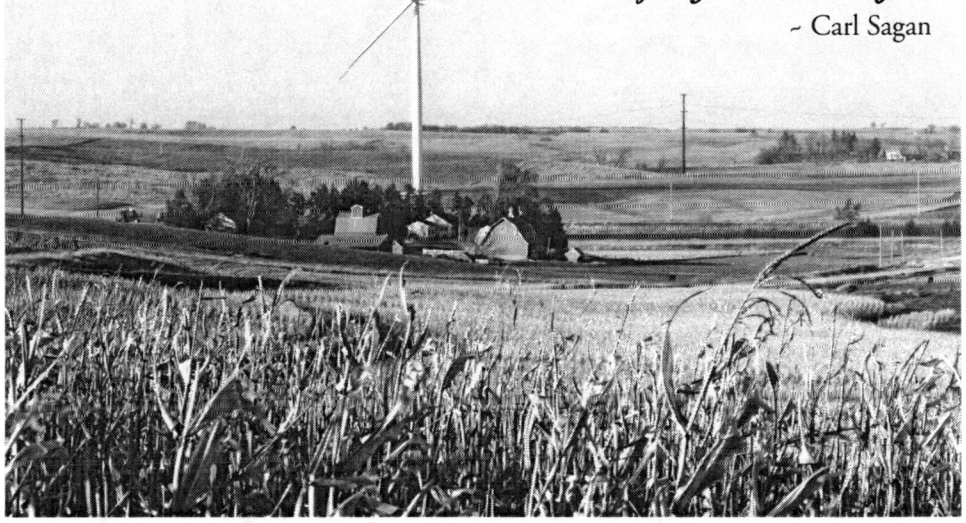

"Science is a way of thinking much more than it is a body of knowledge."

~ Carl Sagan

"Can you smell a rat?" Once you've done a sound check and know what questions to ask, I'd encourage you to try a sniff test. Misinformation, fads, celebrity recommendations, and shoddy science make it tough to find the droplets of facts with the fire hose of information coming at us every day. In short, there are a whole lot of smelly rats out there!

The first check requires considering the credentials of the individual

FOOD CONNECTION POINT 4
Need to find farm and food experts online? We keep lists of food and agricultural experts from around the world.

Farm & Ranch Blogs ~
http://foodconvo.com/SuYSP7
Dietitian Blogs ~
http://foodconvo. com/SPzGWX
Agvocate Blogs ~
http://foodconvo. com/SuYqjY

involved. Does this individual have formal education or professional experience in food or nutrition? For example, consider the nutrition books written by Jillian Michaels, who describes herself as an American personal trainer, reality-show personality, talk-show host, and entrepreneur.

I have no doubt that she's an awesome fitness trainer, but draw the line there. She has no formal education in nutrition (or a college degree), does not adhere to the standards of a registered dietitian (RD) set forth by the Academy of Nutrition and Dietetics (AND), and does not base her food advice in science. In short, she doesn't pass the sniff test.

As Janet Helm, RD, author of the blog Nutrition Unplugged, wrote for MSNBC,[7] "It's easy to be fooled by slim, beautiful actresses who appear to shed pounds as easily as breathing. But their eating regimens are nearly always unnecessarily restrictive. Nutrient deficiencies along with muscle and bone loss are among the risks."

It's no wonder people are confused about food. We see conflicting reports. We hear of different celebrity diets every day while looking for quick fixes to their weight and health problems.

Don't be fooled by anything less than valid science. It's not as sexy, sensational, or emotional as many of the diet and health claims out there, but science is reliable. As the Center for Food Integrity explains, science should be objective. **Science is data driven, repeatable, measurable, and specific.[8]**

Here's a simple litmus test: Does the claim smell like real science? Have you checked the study or only what is reported in the media?

Media bias is a significant concern today, as summarized by former L.A. Times reporter Alisa Valdes:[9] "As one who worked in the belly of the mainstream media beast for nearly a decade, let me explain this phenomenon clearly. For those who make editorial decisions in America's newsrooms, truth is entirely subjective."

Just for the record, one of my degrees required that I take journalism classes. It was pounded into our heads that journalism is not about bias; a journalist's job is to report all angles. This likely won't surprise you, but I was reprimanded more than once for inserting opinion into a piece. I've talked with others holding journalism degrees, and we wonder if those classes are no longer being taught or if journalistic ethics have been thrown out the window by the news industry.

We seem to be on a dangerous path that devalues science and overvalues opinion. Valdes points to a finding from the nonpartisan organization Reporters Without Borders:[10] "Our nation, which has long held 'freedom of the press' to be among our many important liberties, currently ranks 47th in the world for true freedom of the press. With nearly every news outlet owned by just six multinational conglomerates, our editorial content is increasingly controlled (CENSORED) by advertising dollars and internal corporate conflicts of interest."

Valdes noted that in a world where Niger and Estonia rank higher than the United States in press freedoms, we might be smart to ask ourselves the following questions upon reading any news story at all: If this weren't true, who would suffer? If it were true, who stands to benefit?

The following are suggested sites to help you determine what's real science and how to know—particularly when it comes to issues related to farm, food, and nutrition. Please see http://foodconvo.com/VPgZ3a for regular updates to the hyperlinks.

Academics Review

Are you looking at popular claims or at peer-reviewed science? See this site for testing claims.

Registered Dietitian Review of Diet Books

AND spokespeople have reviewed popular diet books to help you understand which diets are reasonable and which should be avoided.

Applied Mythology

What if much that you think you know about agriculture, farming, and food isn't actually true? What if there are "myths" that have been intentionally and mostly unintentionally spread about these issues? This site helps you sort out fact from fiction.

Sense about Science

A charitable trust that equips people to make sense of scientific and medical claims in public discussion.

Biofortified

Volunteer authors provide factual information and foster discussion about agriculture, especially plant genetics and genetic engineering.

Validating Scientific Studies

All of the "junk science" available on the internet makes it critical that we be armed with understanding of what makes a scientific paper truly scientific.

GMO Pundit a.k.a. David Tribe

This site helps readers navigate the confusing myths of modern biology.

Nutrition Guides for Registered Dietitian Practice

Evidence-based guidelines are provided for dietetic and nutrition practitioners to apply research in practice.

Science-Based Medicine

This site explores issues and controversies in the relationship between science and medicine.

International Food Information Council

Great information here effectively communicates science-based information on health, food safety, and nutrition for the public good.

The Journal of Nutrition

Contents include peer-reviewed research reports on all aspects of experimental nutrition.

The Council for Agricultural Science & Technology

Publications written by scientists from many disciplines address issues of animal sciences, food sciences, agricultural technology, and plant & soil sciences.

Food & Drug Administration's Hot Topics in Food Safety

This site covers the FDA's latest information on the hot food safety and nutrition topics.

AND Position Papers (formerly ADA)

Here, the Academy of Nutrition and Dietetics develops Position and Practice Papers to promote the public's optimal nutrition, health, and well-being. The papers written by health professionals who possess thorough and current knowledge of the topic.

Food can kill

Food safety consistently ranks as one of the public's top three concerns about food, so I'm just going to assume it's important to you. After all, who wants to spend their time regurgitating food in the bathroom? I'd like to introduce you to a friend of mine in Tennessee with quite a unique perspective as a doctor that who hears misinformation from patients daily. Samantha E. McLerran, MD, is a mom of three and understands food safety from both sides of the food plate because she's also a beef farmer.

Food safety is a broad and potentially explosive topic. Food safety affects every level of society and every person because we all eat. When I sat down to write, I immediately leapt to my medical roots. Nothing I thought could be more thrilling than a couple of hundred words on food pathogens like E. coli and Salmonella. Yeah, right… my seven year old just rolled her eyes at me and left the room.

"We all eat" is where I started this journey, a statement of an obvious fact. Therefore, food and its safe growth, handling, and processing should be a vital concern of any society. And I will further state that as a society has more and more time and economic resources, they spend more of those assets on food and food development.

When you only get paid $1 for your days work and you spend 50 cents to 75 cents of that dollar on food, you are not going to argue about whether or not it was locally grown and hormone free. If you live in that level of poverty, you don't care if it was produced with biotechnology or from a cloned sheep. You will just be happy to have food there to feed your family so you don't have to listen to your children be hungry and possibly watch them starve to death. You do care that it is sanitary and you hope that it does not carry disease.

Our family is learning about how different farms operate in different parts of the world. One can see how a person's society base influences their perceptions on food safety. Giardia is not a big concern here in the Upper Cumberland (Tennessee), but in third world countries this internal pathogen (stool carried) is a viable threat to your health.

As I read up on statistics and information, I realized Americans are blessed and have no idea on the true impact of the words "food safety." For the most part, the potential food

pathogens that we deal with only make us sick. The CDC estimates that 1 in 6 US citizens will deal with some form of a food borne pathogen each year, with Nor virus being the most common (a.k.a. stomach virus). The hope I, through continued efforts at all levels of the food production chain, preventing these food-borne illness with best practice management practices. 5 million Americans could be prevented from being ill each year if we could decrease the illness load by just 10%. If just one case of E. coli O157 could be prevented, it is estimated the savings could be upwards of several million dollars.

However, there are only 31 known food-borne pathogens which account for 20% of all food-borne illness; the other 80% is caused by unknown or unspecified pathogens. This presents two unique concerns: from a food production standpoint, how do we prevent that which we don't know makes people sick; and then from a medical standpoint, how do we treat what we can't identify?

Beyond these standard food pathogen concerns, we now have to deal with antimicrobial resistance. It is estimated that some strains of Salmonella, Shigella, and some strains of E. coli are rapidly becoming resistant to the antibiotics that are normally used to treat them. These aren't antibiotics from the farm—the resistance is from the people taking them for colds when they don't need them because colds are caused by viruses.

As an American beef producer, home-cookin' mom to three children, and a family practitioner in a small town, I have seen all aspects of food safety. This is a real issue in my day-to-day life from our safe handling practices and animal identification efforts on the farm for ease of tracking of our products, to teaching my kids that you don't cut up raw meat and veggies on the same board and we always wash our hands.

Pathogen	Estimated Number of Hospitalizations	%	Pathogen	Estimated Number of Deaths	%
Salmonella, nontyphoida	19,336	35	Salmonella, nontyphoidal	378	28
Norovirus	14,663	26	Toxoplasma gondii	327	24
Campylobacter spp.	8,463	15	Listeria monocytogene	255	19
Toxoplasma gondii	4,428	8	Norovirus	149	11
E.coli (STEC) O157	2,138	4	Campylobacter spp.	76	6
Subtotal		88	Total		88

The hardest part as a doctor to a patient's family—and the reason this issue will never go away for agriculturists—is that sometimes food-borne pathogens kill. When they or their loved one is ill, I often have little to offer but time, antibiotics, prayer, and a diagnosis of a pathogen that they have only heard about on the news. As the above percentages show,

No More Food Fights!

the 31 known food-borne pathogens account for around 88% of all food-borne-illness-related hospitalizations and deaths. However, that fact is of little comfort to the 12% of Americans that face the unspecified pathogens each year.

My bottom line: Wash your hands after handling raw meat, eat in restaurants you trust, respect the work done by American farmers to bring you one of the safest food-delivery systems on Earth, and don't be quick to blame if there is an outbreak of illness. Sensationalism sells news, but it is not always the truth.

Sensationalism should not trump science!

Samantha raises a good point about the practicality of food safety measures throughout the agrifood system. We have scientific protocol to thank for that safety. It may not be perfect, but we live with an entirely different set of concerns than those in developing countries.

Biotechnology: A bombshell to a civil conversation

One of the most emotionally charged food issues is biotechnology, also known as genetically modified organisms (GMOs) or genetically engineered (GE) organisms. Frankly, this book was partially inspired by the rants of the anti-GMO crowd in the social media world. The trading of insults stands in the face of having a civil conversation, much less one with any meaning.

It seems rather childish that someone should be labeled a prostitute or puppet for big ag just because I believe in the advantages of technology use in farming, but I have been called both. I've also seen companies post innocuous pictures of a breakfast cereal and have a litany of anti-GMO comments on its Facebook page, farmers be verbally attacked for their choice to use biotechnology, and unrelenting grandstanding from both sides.

What's the scoop on biotech? I'd like to introduce you to a scientist friend from Canada, Dr. Cami Ryan. I'm only calling her doctor to be proper; you'd never know she has a PhD on first impression. She's a rodeo-loving mom who lives in beautiful Alberta, Canada, with her family, four horses, and two dogs.

Dr. Ryan is a researcher with the agricultural college at the University of Saskatchewan. She has several peer-reviewed published papers and has worked in the field of biotechnology for almost two decades. She blogs at http://doccamiryan. wordpress.com or you can find her on Twitter @DocCamiRyan. I asked her to explain biotechnology so you can measure it against the sniff test of science for yourself. Just for the record, no one has paid her to say these things.

Man has been changing plants and food for centuries. Brewing beer and making wine and cheese are great examples of this. We do this for many reasons, including to make better quality food and to make farming more productive.

Yes, much has changed over time. The fruits, vegetables, and crops that we see growing today look far different than they did even just a hundred years ago! The great thing is that now we can do things much, much more efficiently. Modern biotechnology[11] is a set of tools and techniques that are applied not only to the development of food and crops but also in many other areas such as medicine, aquaculture, forestry, and even environmental cleanup.

All living matter contains DNA, the "sheet music" for the piano of life. In food and crop production, agricultural technology[12] uses these very tiny bits of living organisms to modify a crop variety or improve a plant's performance. As we discover more about which genes affect different aspects of a plant or crop, scientists can take steps to change that feature or function. In agriculture, this leads to

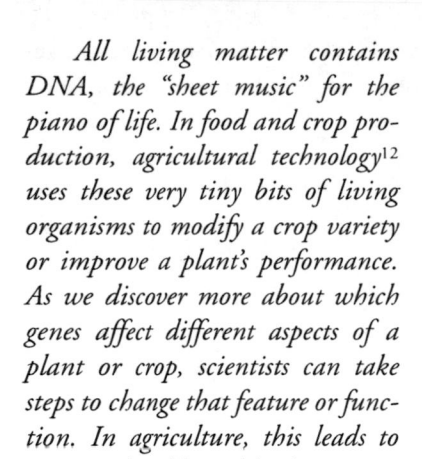

ROTTEN VEGETABLE 6
It is insulting to a farmer to assume they are not making their own choices. I'm not asking you to agree with what they do, but a civil conversation doesn't include accusations of corporate control. Big business and big government and big everything are not the only answers to today's problems. Let's have a deeper discussion.

improved yields and built-in resistances to certain diseases. In other words, scientists can change the notes on the sheet music and improve the piano melody.

Some people think that changing organisms using biotechnology is unnatural. But nothing could be further from the truth. Man has been using far cruder methods for centuries. For example, in the process of cross-breeding all the genes of a plant are introduced to all the genes of another plant. Cross-breeding combines the sheet music for two different songs and then removes the notes that do not sound good, so it's really not that precise. Especially when you consider that modern biotechnology lets scientists choose exactly which genes can be introduced to or changed within the organism.

Let's take a closer look at corn. According to the United States Department of Agriculture (USDA), 80 million acres of land in the US are planted to corn.[13] This corn acreage is used for both human food and animal feed, so it is a very important crop. The European corn borer* was once a serious pest that attacked corn crops throughout the US Corn Belt, devastating family farms and livelihoods. In fact, the corn borer cost the American economy an estimated $1 billion dollars per year! This nasty pest attacks the plant from the inside, eating away at the core of the corn stalk. Conventional pest sprays weren't always effective, as they couldn't reach the pest. Biotechnology had a solution!

A special protein produced by Bacillus thuringiensis (also known as Bt), a naturally occurring soil bacterium, targets corn borers. The tools of biotechnology were used to insert this special protein into Bt corn. The corn now can produce proteins that stop these pests, allowing the corn to survive and thrive. As with any other genetically modified crops, the safety of Bt corn has been thoroughly assessed. It is carefully regulated; academic researchers and national regulatory bodies have concluded that Bt corn is safe for food, for feed, and for the environment.

With the use of modern biotechnology, scientists can transform crop and plant varieties that can be drought-tolerant, ones that can thrive in some of the world's worst growing conditions. Crops can also be made healthier and disease—and pest resistant. Biotechnology can do these things while reducing environmental impact and improving your food. The science of biotechnology holds much promise for helping to feed the world's growing population. And, hey, that's music to my ears!

Genetics have played a big role in the food we consume today. Take a look at the apple bins in your grocery store; there are about 100 varieties grown for commercial

use today as compared to a handful 50 years ago. They were developed for taste and freshness and to meet nutritional needs.

The same can be said for biotechnology, except that biotechnology has been researched far more extensively than the natural genetic selection that's happened over the decades in all types of foods. It's your choice whether you believe in biotech or not; I simply ask you to do a sniff test on peer-reviewed science.

There has been a growing movement to label foods containing any biotech ingredients. Neither the American Medical Association[14], USDA, or FDA has found any science that proves the validity of health concerns, so I find the movement to be far too politically led by the anti-biotech movement. Besides, USDA-certified organic products already offer nearly the same opportunity as what labeling food with biotech ingredients would accomplish. However, I will attempt to explain why labeling is so complicated and expensive.

The first step of tracking biotech products is on the farm, where it needs to be determined if farmers would be required to have different equipment to plant or harvest biotech and non-biotech crops. The most significant concern in the debate is storage. Biotech and non-biotech grain, for example, would not only need separate bins on the farm but would also need to be hauled in different trucks.

The co-op or grain elevator is typically the next place that grain goes. The co-op/elevator would also require different storage for biotech and non-biotech grains. The same would be true for rail cars that haul the grain to the processor. Then, at the processor, different systems or complete sanitation would be necessary to prevent any biotech product residue from entering the non-biotech grains. And for each product derived from grain (corn starch, syrup, corn meal, flour, and oil, for example), there would need to be separation.

The outcome? Food that is more expensive. Some experts estimate $5 billion in costs, but I'm not convinced that anyone really knows. Those costs would be spread across the food system but would ultimately end up in your grocery cart. I don't think it's OK to go to such measures for a practice backed by science, but I will leave that for you to decide in the spirit of a civil conversation.

Do corporations control farmers?

Biotechnology discussions frequently bring up the question "Are big companies, such as Monsanto, Tyson, DuPont, or Smithfield, controlling farmers?" Shake a hand with a farmer and have a conversation; you'll quickly find farmers to be some of the most independent (and stubborn) beings on the face of the earth. The thought of companies controlling them is humorous, at best.

Companies invest decades and millions of dollars in research to develop intellectual property—and then charge accordingly to cover their costs. I'm not going to defend any particular brand, nor will I get in a seed-pricing debate. Seed is expensive, but most technological investments are.

Case in point, Apple's iPhone: The new releases are among the most expensive in the market, yet people line up, camp overnight, and wait to buy the latest release of

a coveted iPhone. I will simply say that businesses with patented products have a right to protect their intellectual property and to sell it according to demand—even if we don't like the products.

In animal agriculture, there are farmers who choose to contract grow for companies because it best fits their families' business models. This doesn't make them any less of farmers; it simply means they have chosen to mitigate some of the risk by contracting to have fixed costs and a set price for the output.

For example, high feed prices and low pork prices results in an $18/head loss for hog farmers. If a farmer typically produces 2,000 hogs per year, that's a $36,000 loss—a clear illustration of why a contract with fixed costs and a guaranteed price might be appealing to a farmer. Some farm families like to contract grow, and others can't stand it—kind of the same as some teachers love teaching and others complaining nonstop.

Let me introduce you to Brian, a farmer I've gotten to know through Twitter. He's a dad to a cute little boy, loves rock 'n' roll concerts, and is a huge fan of a Big 10 school that I refuse to name because it's way too close to our farm. He worked off the farm in retail and then returned home to be a part of the family business. Brian grows corn, soybeans, and popcorn with his father and grandfather. They once raised hogs but went to growing only grains a few years ago because of the pricing I outlined earlier.

Brian also tweets and blogs as The Farmer's Life I highly recommend that you check out his material for a daily perspective from the farm. Brian recently addressed the corporate control of farmers by sharing his entire biotechnology agreement, complete with his commentary:

I've seen a lot of posts online about how corporations control farms or farmers are slaves to "Big Ag." Some people claim that we are beholden to them and have to sign unfair contracts to be privileged enough to use their seed. They'll also claim that the contracts rope us into buying other inputs like pesticides and herbicides from the same company. We get a lot of our seed from big corporations like the "evil" Monsanto, and since Farm Aid seems to be jumping in the debate, I wanted to know what they think about some of the genetically modified crops we grow on our farm.

The Farm Aid website poses the question "What does GE mean for family farmers?" and goes on to say "Corporate Control. Farmers who buy GE seeds must sign contracts that dictate how their crop is grown—including what chemicals to buy—and forbid them from saving seeds. This has given corporations incredible control over the production of major staple crops in America."

Let's examine this corporate control a little further and look at it from the family farm level, my farm in particular. When we buy Monsanto's biotech seeds, we sign a Technology/Stewardship Agreement (which is similar across all companies). Section 4 of the 2011 agreement I have on file covers everything the grower must agree to when purchasing these products. Here's a quick rundown of the requirements.

- *If we buy or lease land that is already seeded with Monsanto technology that year we need to abide by the contract. Makes sense to me. If I end up leasing ground in crop for some reason, I should honor the agreements it was planted with.*

- *Read and follow the <u>Technology Use Guide</u> and <u>Insect Resistance Management/Grower Guide</u>. Monsanto has ideas on how best to use their product. Some of it is required by the EPA to make sure farmers like me understand how to steward the technology. No big surprise there, not to mention that the guides have a ton of good agronomic information.*
- *Implement an Insect Resistance Management program. Shocking! Monsanto thinks controlling pests responsibly is a good idea. If you farm, insects are something you deal with no matter what type of crop you may have.*
- *We should only buy seed from a dealer or seed company licensed by Monsanto. I'd want to do that anyway. It's for my own good. Would you buy a brand new home entertainment system out of the back of some guy's van parked in an alley? Me neither.*
- *We agree to use seed with Monsanto technology solely for planting a single commercial crop. And don't sell any to your neighbor either, it says. That's right, we can't save seed to grow the next year. Frankly I'm not interested in doing that. For the critics who are not sold on biotech crops—do you really want farmers holding onto this seed and planting it without any kind of paper trail?*
- *If you want to plant seed to be used as seed you need to sign an agreement to do so with a seed company licensed by Monsanto. We do this for two different companies. In fact, we've actually worked with one company through several name changes long before biotech showed up. Why? Because we can get a premium price for the soybeans we grow that will be used as seed by other farmers next year.*

We can't grow seed to be used for breeding, research, or generation of herbicide registration data. That gets back to saving seed. If we wanted to breed our own varieties I'm sure we could get into doing that, but I look at it right now as division of labor. Seed companies are great at coming up with great products, and American farmers are the best at turning those products into a bounty of food, feed, fuel, and fiber.

You can see the whole piece, including a PDF of Brian's biotechnology agreement, at http://foodconvo.com/SMKiCt. These agreements are very similar across the various companies that sell biotechnology.

At the end of the day, it's your choice whether you support biotechnology or not, just as it's Brian's choice whether he buys seed with technological improvements and grows it on his farm. I don't think either choice deserves verbal grenades or threats. Do you? I realize there are strong feelings on either end of the spectrum around biotechnology, but let's hold each side accountable to have a more respectful discussion based on science instead of emotion.

I spent five years working in the Reproductive Physiology Laboratory at Michigan State, with glamorous jobs such as washing thousands of pieces of lab glassware, processing mammary glands, and giving cows boluses* in the middle of the night.

Though I was only an undergraduate grunt worker, I took part in rBST trials, melatonin trials, and many others. It gave me a firsthand appreciation for the level of detail that studies require, how dedicated scientists are to their research, and the very lengthy, finite process involved for research to receive government/regulatory approval.

Claiming that scientists sway studies based on funding sources is ridiculous to me. Sure, there are bad apple scientists just as there are poor teachers, parents, farmers, and doctors, but doesn't a scientist ultimately fail in the profession if he or she lacks the ethics to conduct real science? Bad apples are a main reason for, the value of peer-reviewed science—and taking time to be diligent in checking how research weighs against popular opinion.

Be aware of articles stilted one way, and get answers from those with first-hand expertise in the food system. A journalist using shoddy science as his or her singular source to push opinion isn't an expert, and neither is a celebrity who became a food diva or the top search result on Google. Nor are books like *Skinny Bitch*, which push extreme viewpoints that mess with people's minds.

Experts can be found in the scientists researching inputs, farmers producing raw products, processors making it the raw products into food, and registered dietitians who have studied how food impacts human nutrition.

Remember the sense of smell; do food claims pass the sniff test of science, or do they reek of sensationalism and celebrity? Check it out with those in the know!

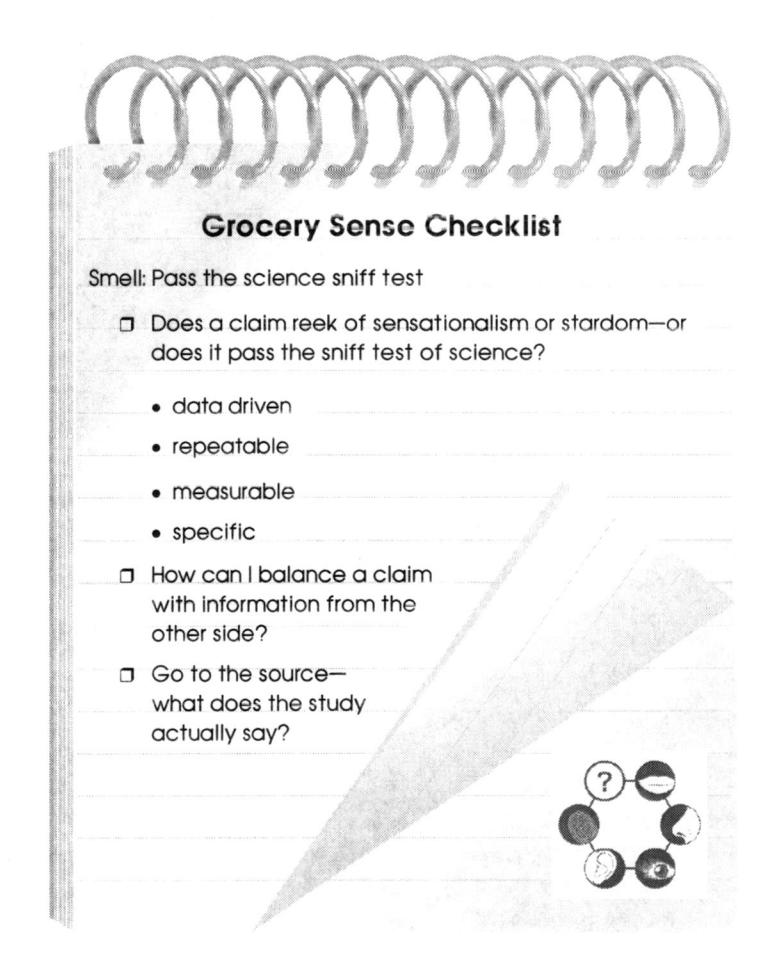

Grocery Sense Checklist

Smell: Pass the science sniff test

☐ Does a claim reek of sensationalism or stardom—or does it pass the sniff test of science?

- data driven
- repeatable
- measurable
- specific

☐ How can I balance a claim with information from the other side?

☐ Go to the source— what does the study actually say?

Taste: Do You Feel Good About Your Personal Choice?

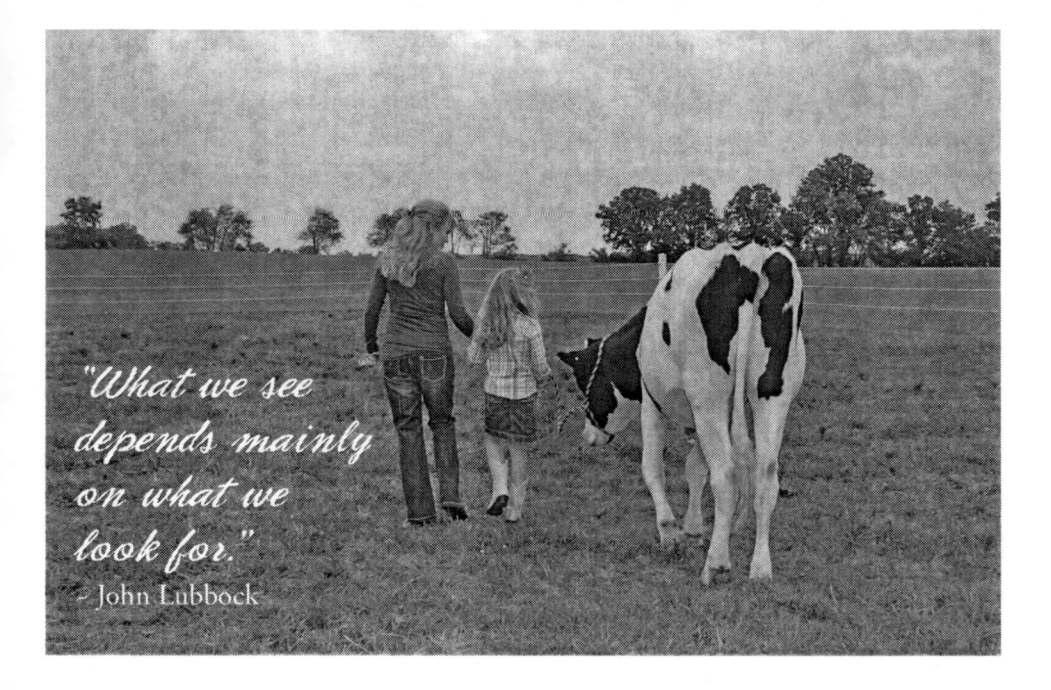

"What we see depends mainly on what we look for."
~ John Lubbock

"Is it O.K. to feed my little girl regular milk?" asked my friend, Kim, while we were relaxing on a sailboat watching the sun set over Lake Michigan on a beautiful September evening. We were wrapping up a professional development event, so I inquired why she was asking. "I'm overwhelmed, confused and frustrated with all of the milk labels! Should I feel guilty if I don't buy the expensive stuff that labeled organic, hormone and antibiotic free?" I explained it was a matter of taste—and knowing the facts.

Taste and food go hand-in-hand, right? Your taste may tend toward the gourmet side, while your friend might be a meat-and-potatoes guy. Is one person wrong for his or her personal taste? Is grass-fed meat really better? Is organic the only way to

> **ROTTEN VEGETABLE 7**
> **Label versus logic.**
> Consider this; all food has hormones in it (it always has). An argument could be made that most food is natural and that bucolic images on certain brands don't always represent reality. Labels are marketing tools; don't let their claims overcome your logic.

go? Is there really such a thing as hormone-free food? Am I a bad parent if I'm not purchasing the foods that marketing is guilting me into?

NO! It's a simple answer, perhaps too simple for some, yet I talk to mothers every day who worry about if they're doing the right things for their families when they select food at the grocery store. Author David Ropier points out in *How Risky Is It, Really?* "The less we know, the more afraid we are likely to be."[15]

We have fewer people involved with farming and many, many food activists trying to sway opinions. This adds up to people being afraid—and I believe *all* sides of the food plate have a responsibility to work together to provide open, accurate information. That means farmers can't hide behind our technical jargon, scientists have to get out of the lab, and dietitians must find ways to explain what they do.

Again, food doesn't have to be complicated, and it should not involve guilt. It's a personal choice. Some people have to make their choice on economics. Others buy based on labels. Nutrition is the key concern for some. Still others shop at only certain stores.

FOOD CONNECTION POINT 5
Who is responsible for the obesity epidemic? The people growing and processing food, those marketing it, or the individuals putting it in their mouths? Personal responsibility is something that the farm side of the food plate takes pretty seriously. It might be common ground.

The FDA and USDA maintain extensive standards to ensure that our food is safe. These organizations are not perfect, but they do monitor, test, and regulate what happens across the agrifood system (you can read more about that later in the chapter).

Case in point, milk: All Grade A milk—the only variety sold in grocery stores in the United States—is antibiotic free. Even the stuff without the label proclaiming it's antibiotic free (and usually two times the price). The USDA makes sure of this, and farmers take it pretty seriously, as my friend Joanne will explain in a bit.

Overcoming food guilt

As mentioned in the first paragraph of this chapter, Kim was guilt-ridden as she tried to find the balance between her family's health and their budget. She wrote about her experience and the guilt associated with mom's making food choices in the grocery store..

Is it possible to go to the grocery store without being confused and then overwhelmed by guilt around food? We learned talking to people in agriculture can help with that.

Being the mom of a curly haired little girl, I have spent the last two and a half years being inundated with what I think is "fear-based marketing" about nutrition for myself, when I was pregnant, and for my growing cherub.

In our line of work, my husband and I try extra hard to live a stress-free lifestyle and all of the messages I was receiving about nutrition were really stressing me out. Talk about Adultitis™![16]

Being self-employed and in charge of marketing for our company, I am conscious of how "fear-based marketing" works. It really stinks to be on the consumer side of such fear tactics.

Through blogs, parenting sites, T.V. shows, Facebook, and just hearing others [sic] moms talking, true or not—this is the message I heard loud and clear…

"Do not buy 'regular milk' for your one year-old. Do you know what's in there? You need to bite the bullet financially and go organic—for the health and well-being of your child."

Well, I bought the "regular" milk anyway and hoped the fear-based marketing was just a ploy to sell overpriced milk. But was it?

You can find Kim's full discussion at http://foodconvo.com/PDUekw. As Kim and I talked about how confusing food could be, I explained that milk isn't causing girls to have to wear bras in the second grade and that no milk has antibiotics in it. All food has hormones in it—including the food you ate for lunch and that which you shoved into your mouth as a toddler.

Are food labels a game of Truth or Dare?

It would be great to get Kim and Joanne, another mom friend of mine, together, but maybe they'll meet through this book. Joanne didn't grow up on a farm, but she knew from spending time with her grandpa that she loved cows. She's a Cornell graduate, works in ag financing and fell in love with a man who also wanted to milk cows, so they're slowly building their herd.

They're now living in upstate Vermont, milking 30 little brown cows (Jerseys) and growing their family. Joanne also blogs because she believes in dairy farmers, regardless of size or type of farm, and was asked to write a guest post for a mommy blogger at http://foodconvo.com/T1E0Se.

My guess is that as you approach our farm and see our girls grazing our rolling green hills in Northeast Vermont, you would maybe assume we are an organic* herd. We are not, and I will get into the why not at the end of this post.

The average price of a gallon of "conventional"* whole milk was $3.63 in March 2012. Organic milk was $4.02 per half-gallon or $8.04 per gallon[17] I wanted to get those figures out there so we know exactly what we're talking about a cost that's more than double. If you're a family of five and buying five gallons a week, those dollars add up fast. Is the added expense worth it?

If you ask me, I'd say no. Of course I would—we produce milk that is not organic. But I know there are some people who choose the certified organic label for other items and extend that preference to milk, which is their choice. But in my opinion, I think it's irresponsible to make people feel guilty if they don't want to or can't shell out the extra cash for the label without an adequate explanation, especially when budgets are tight.

When companies sell products, they're obviously looking for an edge. This comes in the form of price or quality, for example, but ultimately their edge is based on consumer perception. Labels and other retail packaging are often used to convey a claim to alter the perception of the product in order to sell more or to sell at a higher price. This often leaves products without special labels looking somehow inferior with no adequate explanation. It underscores the importance for food and nutrition professionals to communicate science-based facts about food.

So then, what does the certified organic label on milk mean and why is it so much more expensive?

Milk is Milk

There is no significant difference in the composition of milk that comes from cows that are raised with organic practices or those that are from conventional farms.[18] *The same nutrients and hormones exist in both, both are safe to consume and BOTH are free from antibiotics. Interesting to note, there is no way to test milk to determine whether it was from an organic farm or a conventional farm—or one that uses rBST or one that does not. Bottom line, milk is milk.*

Because of the combination of nine essential nutrients, milk—organic or otherwise—packs a powerful punch for a healthy diet. The USDA and the U.S. National Academy of Sciences define an essential nutrient as a dietary substance required for healthy body functioning. The nine found in milk are: Calcium, Potassium, Phosphorus, Protein, Vitamin D, Vitamin A, Vitamin B12, Riboflavin and Niacin. Sometimes, there can be a very slight difference in fat and protein levels between organic and conventional milk, but this is thought to have more to do with the cows' diet than any other factor.[19] *You might see this same difference in milk amongst different brands or from a local, seasonally grazed herd that may or may not be organic.*

When it comes to safety, all milk sold in stores is processed to kill harmful bacteria—either through pasteurization or ultra-high temperature processing. However, milk, along with many other food products, is not a sterile product and thus some tolerance is allowed for bacteria counts. In a study examining the composition of milk from organic and conventional farms, the bacteria counts were lower in conventionally labeled milk.[20] *However, the difference was minimal, and both were far below the federal limit.*

Along those same lines, hormones are present in all milk—organic, rBST-free, conventional, chocolate, strawberry, coffee, skim, 2%, etc. The same study found a few small differences in hormone levels between conventional and organic milk. While organic milk was slightly lower in IGF-1, it had higher progesterone and estrogen concentrations than conventional milk. However, these differences are not likely to be biologically significant in humans consuming organic or conventional milk.

Finally to be absolutely clear, all milk on the shelf in the grocery store is free of antibiotics. Taking it a step further, organic farmers pledge not to use antibiotics on their cattle.[21] *If they do, the cow must leave the herd. On a conventional farm, the farmer is allowed to use antibiotics to treat a sick cow. However, the milk she produces is withheld from mixing with the rest of the herd's until it is tested and shown to be clear of the antibiotic. Many tests are done on the milk in its journey from farm to store shelf to ensure that there are no antibiotics present. The farmer risks losing his/her license to sell milk if antibiotics are found. This is not an area where farmers like to mess around!*

You can tell Joanne cares deeply about her cows and the milk they produce, and that people understand what they're buying based on labels. You may think her little farm sounds idyllic, but check out her blog at http://farmlifelove.com to get a perspective on the value of large farms.

As of the writing of this book, dairy farmers of all sizes are suffering from low milk prices and record high feed prices from the drought. Many are operating in the red and take home about a quarter ($0.25) per gallon you pay in the store because of an outdated milk-pricing system. This situation is also a pretty clear indicator that farmers like Joanne must love what they do.

There are many different tastes for food, just as there are many different ways to farm. Let's not judge each other based on our labels of choice; instead, let's gain perspective to appreciate the true differences in our food choices.

Does your hamburger cause global warming?

We are exposed to thousands of marketing messages a day, and it seems like a disproportionate number of those are associated with food. Food guilt trips drive me crazy, as you likely figured out in my grocery store introduction. You can also see on my post at http://foodconvo.com/ZnO6Qb about Cheetos being required on our family vacations.

Some food marketing messages are particularly laden with guilt. Case in point: eat less meat to save the environment. Some USDA figures shows that the average Americans are under-consuming protein—and I'm likely one of those. I love salad. I have plenty of meatless days and survive.

That's my choice, not a guilt trip promoted by animal rights activists. I'd encourage you to get the real science before you are guilted into Meatless Monday or into feeling "less green" when you consume meat. Frankly, the Meatless Monday messages (started by the very questionable Environmental Working Group,[22] amongst others) make me feel green—and not in the environmental way.

Dr. Jude Capper, PhD, http://bovidiva.com, is proudly British but has done extensive research on livestock's environmental impact at Washington State and Cornell Universities. She also has great appreciation for fine food, good cooking, and wine. Jude brings an expert perspective on improvements in animal agriculture that have led to a reduced environmental impact of eating meat.

Do we need to moderate meat consumption in order to feed the world in 2050? Given beef producers' track record of ingenuity, it's possible but not probable. Is it possible to supply nine billion people with 250 pounds of meat per capita in 2050?

The question stemmed from a recent paper[23] in which Stockholm scientists claimed that we would all have to reduce meat consumption by 75% by 2050 in order to have enough water to supply the population. Then there was subsequent rebuttal[24] from the American Society of Animal Science—in which several scientists noted the flaws in the Swedish paper, the importance of animal proteins in the diet and the use of marginal land for grazing livestock.

On Twitter, the comment[25] was made that there appear to be two distinct sides to this argument— one side (the environmentalists and anti-animal agriculture groups) warning that we need to drastically cut meat consumption in order to feed everybody—and the other (the meat industry) turning a blind eye and effectively promoting the idea that we can eat all the meat that we like without having any environmental impact.

We're nowhere near 250-pound meat consumption per capita globally. Even U.S. consumers who are often portrayed as meat-guzzling bacon-o-philes have an average annual consumption of 171 pounds[26] according to the USDA.[27] As current beef consumption is 58 pounds/person in the US, that's a lot of pork and chicken that will presumably make up the difference.

Beef production uses considerable amounts of land and water, but should we expect producers to effectively shoot themselves in the foot and suggest that consumers forgo a cheeseburger in favor of an alfalfa sprout salad? Isn't improved efficiency a characteristic of every successful industry?

The motor industry is a major contributor to environmental concerns, yet automobile manufacturers aren't saying "we're going to produce cars in the same way that we did in the '50s, you'll just have to drive less." Instead, the message is something akin to "we're making cars more energy-efficient so that you can continue to drive without worrying about your car's environmental impact."

That's exactly what the beef industry has done, is doing and will continue to do into the future. Since 1977, the US beef industry has cut water use by 12%, land use by 33% and the carbon footprint of one pound of beef by 16%. Providing that producers are still able to use management practices and technologies that improve efficiency, further reductions should be seen in future.

So do we need to moderate meat consumption in order to feed the world in 2050? I'd love to be able to answer this by citing a published paper that has taken improvements in meat industry productivity over the next 40 years into account rather than assuming a "business as normal" outcome. In the absence of such a paper, I'll simply point to beef producers' track record of ingenuity, it's possible but not probable.

Globally, there are huge opportunities for improved efficiency and concurrent reductions in resource use from all meat production systems—the key is not to reduce meat production but simply to produce it more efficiently.

You choose what the environmental standard is for your food, but please know that there is decreasing carbon footprint from animal agriculture. Personally, I believe people have the right to select hamburgers, pork chops and chicken breasts any day because the nutrition easily outweighs the environmental impact.

Excuse me, there's a germ in my food

Food safety is a shared responsibility. It begins before the first seed is planted or animal is birthed—and ends when the food is in your stomach. If you've ever suffered from food poisoning, you know how miserable it can be when one part of the system is broken.

Blame might lie with a wild animal urinating on vegetables (as has happened with recalls), a farmer not following protocol, a processor who is neglectful, a grocer who didn't cool products properly or a germ-filled cutting board in your kitchen.

The protocols in place protect food until it arrives in your kitchen makes me feel good about our food, but studies show that the majority of you don't believe it's as safe as it was when you were growing up.[28] There are likely many reasons, so I'll simply offer a good source for information.

The International Food Information Council, one of my favorite sources for unbiased information, has an excellent description of the federal food system in the United States—you can find more at http://foodconvo.com/PSbzGD. Just don't let the acronyms intimidate you!

From the corn farmer to the poultry processor to our favorite grocer or restaurant, all are important links in our shared responsibility to ensure a safe and abundant food supply. To maintain our status as a leader in ensuring safe food, our food-production system is highly regulated by laws and guidance ensure that everyone producing food fulfills his or her responsibility to maintain the safety levels.

Food-chain producers, processors, and manufacturers are primarily responsible for ensuring the safety of our food supply; the FDA and the USDA are responsible for oversight. They work together and are interconnected with state and local partners, farmers and producers, the food industry, retailers, and food—service establishments to provide oversight on the safety of food in the United States.

US Food and Drug Administration (FDA)

In the United States, the FDA regulates approximately 80% of our food supply. The FDA is also responsible for protecting public health by advancing innovations to make food safer and affordable. The FDA also ensures that food products are labeled correctly and truthfully to appropriately inform consumers.

In addition, the FDA develops standards for food ingredients, colors, and additives. It conducts research to detect and identify potential contaminants in food—whether naturally occurring or from man-made sources such as packaging. The agency also inspects food—processing plants, imported food products, and animal food facilities.

The Food Safety Modernization Act (FSMA) is the most historic piece of food-safety legislation passed by Congress since the enactment of the Food, Drug and Cosmetic Act (FDCA) of 1938, which gave the FDA the authority to oversee the safety of food, drugs, and cosmetics. The Food Safety Modernization Act of 2011 is hailed as historic because it focuses on prevention and provides the FDA with tools and with inspection and enforcement authority to ensure that unsafe foods are not available to the public.

In addition to tools such as increased records inspection and the authority to deny entry, the FSMA also provides the FDA with mandatory recall authority. In lieu of relying on a firm's voluntary decision to remove suspected food from the marketplace, the FDA can now order a mandatory recall of such products if there is evidence the food is adulterated or misbranded or can be a danger to public health. The FDA has also launched a new consumer search engine where news and information about the latest recalls are posted and updated regularly.

US Department of Agriculture (USDA)

The USDA's Food Safety and Inspection Service (FSIS) is the public-health arm of the USDA that ensures the safety of meat, poultry, and egg products. The FSIS ensures that

these products are properly inspected, labeled, and packaged. The FSIS also monitors raw meat and poultry products for bacterial contamination, drug residues, and other chemicals. An interconnected network of other agencies and departments also works continuously to ensure a safe and abundant food supply.

Producers, government, manufacturers, and retailers are required by law to apply food—safety standards at every point along the food chain, except one—in your home.

Farmers work to feed hungry mouths around the globe

One of the perspectives you'll likely hear a lot about from the agriculture side is the need to feed world—an obvious disconnect when studies show that 40% of food buyers don't think it's the job of the United States to provide food for other countries.[29] Yet it's an area of high priority to the farm side of the plate, as our global population is expected to reach 9 billion people by 2050 and 1 billion people are currently living in food insecurity.[30]

The eyes of a hungry child will forever be seared into my heart after seeing millions live in poverty in South Africa. When I volunteer at our local school, I see hungry children who can't learn until they're fed breakfast. Both are sad truths, albeit two very different situations.

The majority of residents in developed countries aren't facing starvation, but finding nutrition is a daily challenge for more kids than you might realize. The white paper *"Making Safe, Affordable, Abundant Food a Global Reality"* reports that the problem of childhood poverty and hunger is very real to:

- 2 of 5 children living in inner London
- 1 of 8 children in France
- 1 of every 7 children in Japan
- 1 in every 5 children in the United States

Nearly 3 billion people—almost 43% of the world's population—currently live on less than $2 US/day, reports UNICEF. In the world's poorest countries, citizens can spend from 50% to 80% of their income on food.[31]

Working in developing countries such as Egypt and the Ukraine gave me a first-hand view of challenges related to politics, infrastructure, and tradition in agriculture. It would be ideal to teach people in other countries how to farm, helping them learn techniques to grow and safely process foods. I agree that should be the objective, but I also know what happens when "foreign trainers" go home and politics, economics, and infrastructure challenges become a daily reality. Unfortunately, the answer isn't as simple as "teach a man to fish…"

In short, when there are hungry people in need of food, it's really hard to for people on the farming side of the plate to turn their backs. Some will claim food insecurity is all about infrastructure and distribution, but I don't believe that's the case. Food security a complex problem: part of the answer is found in Canadian and American food production.

Agriculture has the capability; therefore, they shoulder the responsibility. It's a choice that helps farmers feel good about their work. It may not be an area you think about every day, but farmers do—and would like to talk about it with you.

There are many perspectives and choices in the global discussion around food. Rest easy knowing there is a long-standing, closely monitored, and often updated system in place to provide you with safe, abundant food.

Just as your kitchen isn't likely to be 100% germ-free, the agrifood system isn't perfect. However, the system involves a lot more science and inspections than that thing growing at the back of my refrigerator (and yes, food waste is a part of the food discussion).

While we're working on the tough global issues, let's celebrate having safe, abundant food choice for our families. It's something my family gives thanks for at each meal and I hope you will, too.

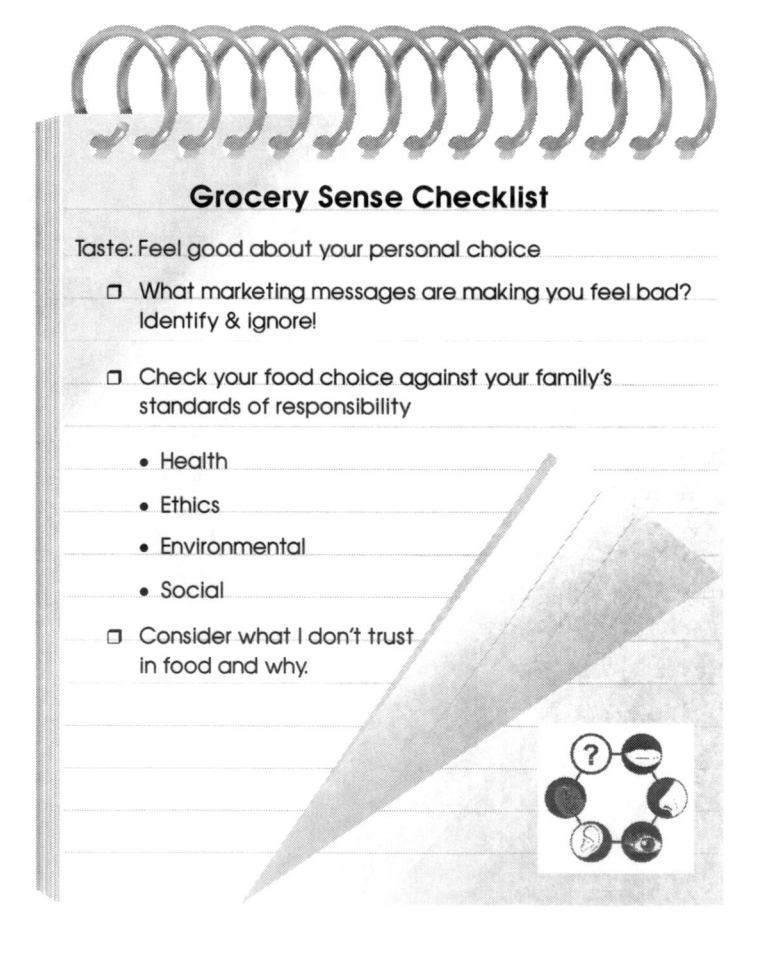

Grocery Sense Checklist

Taste: Feel good about your personal choice

- ☐ What marketing messages are making you feel bad? Identify & ignore!

- ☐ Check your food choice against your family's standards of responsibility

  - Health
  - Ethics
  - Environmental
  - Social

- ☐ Consider what I don't trust in food and why.

Common Sense: Remember the Basics!

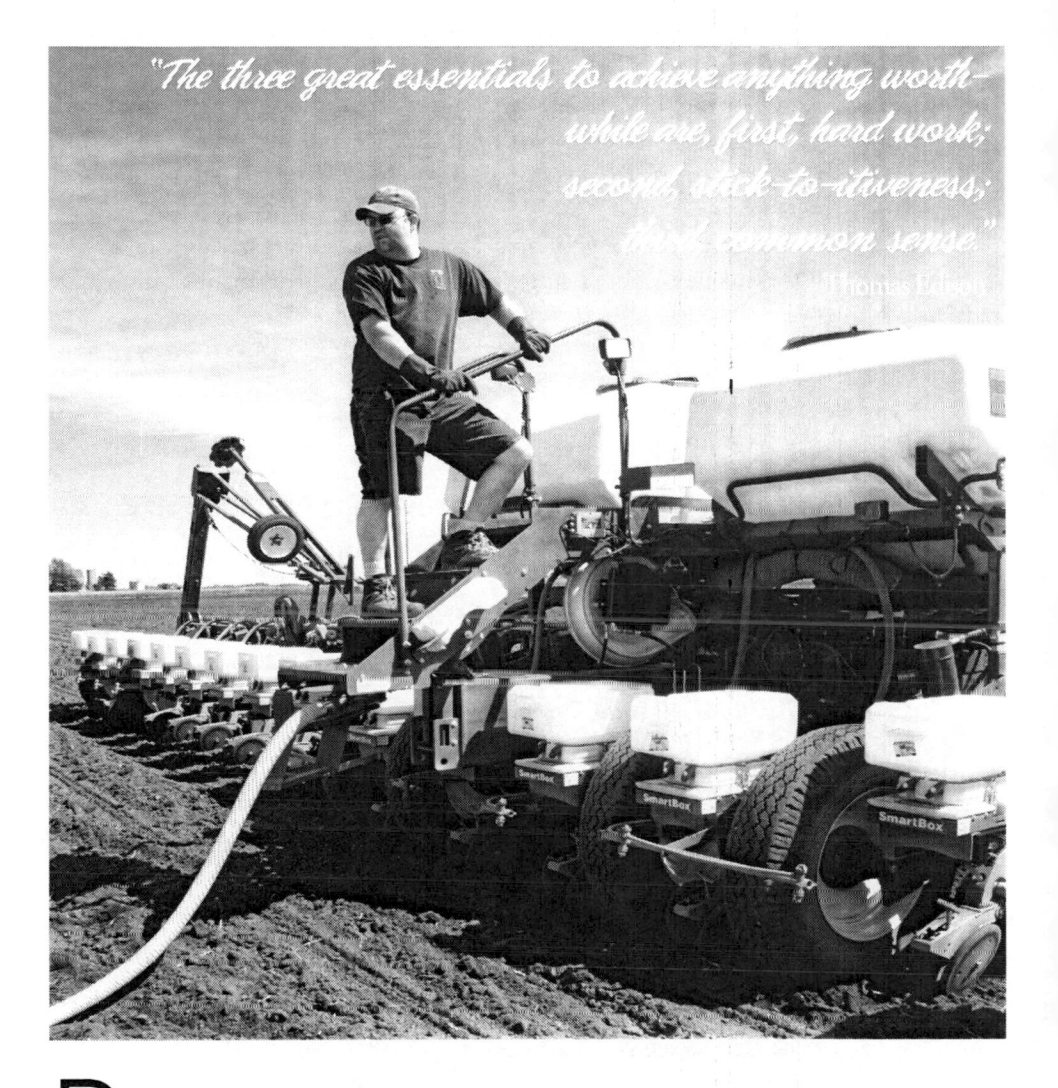

"The three great essentials to achieve anything worth-while are, first, hard work; second, stick-to-itiveness; third, common sense."

—Thomas Edison

Remember when your grandma fed you cookies, when you inhaled food in college because you were so grateful to have more than noodles in a package, and when macaroni and cheese was a gourmet delight? You enjoyed it because it was good and you were hungry. Food is a basic necessity, and in a land of overabundance, we seem to lose sight of that.

An International Consumer Attitude Survey showed that 95% of consumers buy food on taste, price, and nutrition. So let's not have the conversation clouded by politics and propaganda. Good food that is affordable and nutritious is a shared goal around the plate, right?

Common sense tells us that there many different ways to accomplish good food that doesn't cost an arm and a leg. Rhetoric and regulations drive costs up for all of us, so let's take a look at a few of the key issues we haven't already tackled to find some reason.

Is local really the most sustainable?

Local food makes sense, right? Food that's grown closer tastes better, travels fewer miles, and supports the community. My family likes to grow our own veggies, buy beef from a friend, pick fruit locally, and we are quite partial to Michigan's red haven peaches and Indiana's cantaloupes. However, my family also enjoys bananas, almonds from California, and fresh fruits in the winter.

Eating local food seems like common sense, until you read *The 'Locavores Dilemma: In Praise of the 10,000-mile Diet*. If you're into food, I recommend the book—though I warn you to prepare yourself for a very cerebral read. Authors Desrochers and Shimizu summarize **"Turning our back on the global food supply chain, and in the process, reducing the quantity of food produced in the most suitable locations will inevitably result in larger amounts of inferior land being put under cultivation."**[32]

They go on to point to lower yields and greater environmental damage, as well as the locavores' rejection of technological advancements such as no-till farming* (a practice several farmers

> **FOOD CONNECTION POINT 6**
> Look at a farm as a large garden. You know those nasty aphids on your roses or tomatoes? Or, if you're like our family, you have squash beetles that literally suck the life out of your pumpkins. Ugh. Food doesn't grow without pests associated—bugs (and worms) have to eat too. Food production requires pest control —even "organic" and "natural" farming.
>
> Do you have garden markers you're especially proud of? The signs at the ends of fields are like big garden markers—they are to mark the type of seed that's planted, which includes the company the seed was purchased from and which variety it is. Those signs are not real estate or ownership signs as some studies show that non-farm people think. Field signs are "garden markers" that allow comparisons between seed varieties.
>
> Farming can be similar to many activities you're involved with, once you take a closer look. What other examples can you think of?

have referenced in No More Food Fights!). The authors also share numerous life cycle assessment studies that have "debunked" locavores' claims about greenhouse gases associated with food miles. As it turns out, **producing food requires a lot more energy than transporting food, particularly if heating or cool of the products is necessary during transport.**

For example, shipping freshly picked apples from New Zealand in that country's summer to the United Kingdom during its winter is actually more sustainable because less energy is used in cold storage. Apples grown in the United Kingdom and stored for five to nine months (experiencing normal food loss rates) used 8%-16% more energy in studies cited in *The Locavores Dilemma..*

The Locavore's Dilemma is too complex to write about in full detail, but to quote the authors on the myth of locavorism healing the earth: "A world with modern agriculture will dramatically curtail our impact on the environment. Increased competitive pressures cause farmers to constantly find new and better ways of doing things, including economies of scale, relocating their operations or increasing their purchases from businesses located in more suitable areas—which will spare nature while increasing production."

That seems like common sense to the farm side of the plate, but I'm curious—does it seem that way to the food side? Food and sustainability expert Ronald Bailey from Reason.com says that the "debate over the food miles is a distraction from the real issues that confront global food production."[33]

Integrity and expertise in humane animal care

Before you chalk this section up to another farm person who doesn't value animals as much as you do, consider this: I have shed thousands of tears about my cows dying, given them IVs with more love than the hospital gives humans, supported baby calves who could not stand, nurtured kittens from near death, watched my 4-H animals be loaded onto trailers for slaughter, and I still remember the heartbreak of my first cat getting run over by a UPS truck.

I've also had my body implanted into the side of a truck by an irate dairy heifer (yes, I left a dent), been cornered by a protective mother cow, and had a cow flip me up over a free stall*, slammed on the metal bar on my back.

In short, I understand animals. I love them, even when they're rotten. **I believe animals should receive the best possible care and be treated with respect.** However, as a farmer, I know animals are not human and should not be valued the same as humans. Common sense says that Sweetie the cat does not have the same value as Sweetie our child.

Farm animals, as much as we may love them, serve a purpose. That purpose is to provide food for humans. And it is farmers' privilege to care for animals so they can fulfill that role. It seems as though many people get squeamish talking about that the life cycle, but remember—my cow is not your dog. One is for sustenance and the other for companionship, but both deserve to be treated with respect; that is just common sense.

Imagine this: You hire a babysitter to come into your home and care for your children. Two weeks after the seemingly qualified babysitter was in your home, you find videos posted on YouTube, your family's name smeared across newspaper headlines, your home on the nightly news, and people glaring at you as you walk down the street.

The video's content? You—spanking your child in an act of discipline. Would you feel as though your privacy had been intruded upon just because the babysitter didn't agree with your methodology (and had never discussed this with you)? Would the babysitter's secret videotaping be seen as an act of integrity? Likely not.

Hidden videotaping on a farm is no different. A farmer's feelings about being portrayed as someone who "abuses" animals are the same that you'd feel if a babysitter used a hidden camera in a writing pen to videotape you "abusing" a child in the spanking scenario. Both hidden videos are an invasion of privacy, neither is an

appropriate response, and such behavior reeks of sensationalism. Moreover, if true abuse is happening, it should be reported immediately to the authorities, not compiled into a viral video with dramatic music.

Should a farm operate as a business with the expectation that all people caring for animals conduct themselves with integrity? Yes! Do animals deserve to be treated with respect for the sacrifice they make to provide us with food? Absolutely. Is it fair to label farmers as lacking animal-care standards because of a few bad actors? No.

The fact that farmers respect their animals contradicts what many animal-rights activists want you to believe. Some are polished smooth-talkers like Wayne Pacelle of HSUS and more radical groups damage property and/or people. I saw extremist groups attempt to burn down the animal science building and blow up Agriculture Hall at MSU. Frankly, farm families live in fear of such tactics by animal rights and environmental activists, just as you would if your family home and business were terrorized.

This fear can hinder farmers from interacting with you, as animal agriculture practices can look terrible, even when considered a "best management practice" or one done in the best interest of the animal. It so frustrating to us—and never far from mind, even when there's emergencies with animals.

My close friend Kelly, who milks our cows, called me on a sticky 90-degree day, in August with an unusually stressed voice. "I just found Princess down in the pasture. Can you come help?" Princess, obviously named by our daughter, is one of the cows my husband and I own. As I raced over to the lush green pasture, I saw Princess laying stretched out and not in great shape—she appeared to have been down (unable to stand) for several hours in the heat and was laboring to breathe.

"I'll go get the tractor if you stay with her" said Kelly. She hurried off to the barn to get the tractor while I focused on keeping Princess alive. This required me smacking her across the face and kneeing her chest as hard as my human weight could muster.

Before you judge me; consider the shock it takes to keep a human heart going— and then multiply that by 10. Kelly returned with the necessary heavy equipment; we got Princess up by putting a metal device known as a hip lift around her hip bones as Kelly raised the hip lift with the tractor and I provided leverage on the halter so Princess could stand.

As we waited for her to become steady enough to walk, Kelly and I talked about how terrible the incident would look on video if captured by animal rights activists. We helped Princess back to the barn with Kelly carefully driving the tractor and the hip lifts holding Princess up as I kept her steady on the halter. It was not a pretty scene; urine was pouring out of the cow and there was manure was everywhere (cows don't use bedpans).

Is this an image we want on camera? I think not. It would look terrible on the nightly news and could be incorrectly labeled as animal abuse, yet the cow lived and did not suffer needlessly—because two women cared enough to do some ugly things in the interest of animal welfare.

Unfortunately, the fear of being unfairly portrayed by animal rights activists is very real in the farming world, and it can keep farmers from reaching across the plate. You can see why by reading more about the activists.

Sarah Hubbart has a picture of her dog Hobbes on her Facebook page, is a self-confessed foodie, and brings a great deal of personal passion to correcting the misperceptions of animal welfare, along with pursuing this correction professionally.

She learned about the animal rights movement firsthand in Washington, DC. She fits the urbanite mold pretty well in DC, but the truth is that she's a farm girl from California. Sarah has attended animal rights conferences, discussed the movement as a part of her master's degree work, and observed the movement's efforts firsthand. She has this to say:

Back in 1987, the dawn of the animal rights movement in the United States, a group of activist leaders assembled to create the first-ever animal rights caucus and with it, a manifesto for their new cause. Their "Animal Rights Agenda" included one particularly bold action item: "We call for the eventual elimination of animal agriculture."

That may sound laughable or perhaps impossible. But in the past decade, these extreme animal rights groups have capitalized on the urban-rural disconnect and the rise of the Internet to expand their influence.

They have enjoyed political and financial success by demonizing farmers and their practices. They use emotional, and often blatantly false, terminology while describing modern farms as places where chickens are "crammed in cages" or pigs are "pumped full of drugs."

And make no mistake—they do have one goal in mind. The eradication of livestock production altogether. They realize that this is a slow, incremental process. And that's why we all must understand the threat these extreme groups represent.

Most animal rights activist campaigns hinge on making the public feel guilty about eating meat. Some speakers at the 2012 National Animal Rights Conference compared poultry farms with the Holocaust's concentration camps; others compared their efforts to promote animal rights with the civil rights movement. A few speakers promoted illegal activity and reassured attendees that going to jail for the cause is "worth it."

I've realized that although the terms "animal rights" and "animal welfare" are often used interchangeably by both activists and those in agriculture, it is clear that they do not mean the same thing! And the things that many activists say about farmers and farming couldn't be further from the truth.

The farmers and ranchers I know work hard to ensure the welfare of their animals. Getting up at 2 a.m. to check on a newborn calf embodies what "animal welfare" means to me. Animal rights, on the other hand, follows the extreme ideology that animals are not ours to use for any purpose, be it food, companionship, or otherwise. Obviously, that does not align with the values of most Americans.

I've also learned that things are not always as they seem. For example, the HSUS is not affiliated with local humane societies (or any animal shelter, and only 6% of members of the Physicians Committee for Responsible Medicine are actually doctors (but the group was founded by the notoriously extreme group PETA). These organizations rely on the misperception that they represent a mainstream, commonsense view to promote a very extreme agenda.

Thankfully, the ideologies of vocal activist groups do not reflect the values of most Americans. As a nation, 97% of us enjoy meat, milk, and eggs—we just want to feel good about that choice. And it seems like common sense to me that you should! I believe in

agriculture, and I believe in our nation's farmers, and I think that today's livestock producers should be proud of the important work that they do.

My hope is that farmers and their customers can continue to build an ongoing dialogue about modern animal agriculture that is based on fact and not just emotion.

If you'd like to know more about the animal rights movement, connect with Sarah at @MustBeSarah on Twitter. I hope her perspective has provided a dose of common sense about animal rights activists and about farmers' commitments to animal welfare.

Why grass can't feed an Olympian

Let's compare a bovine to an Olympian to get a bit of insight about the technical care of farm animals. Not to suggest a cow as a torchbearer at the next Olympics, though cattle are pretty fast when they decide to be ornery (it's quite irritating to be outrun by a 1,500-pound beast you're trying to help). As my PhD dairy nutritionist friend Robin penned, a lactating dairy cow has a high metabolism and is very similar to a marathon runner or high-performance athlete:

"Cows need nutritionists?" is the response that I frequently get from family members and fellow travelers in airports, when they ask about my work. Many people still think that dairy cows consume grass and grass alone. They have that idyllic image of black and white cows out in a green pasture next to a red barn. While some cows can sustain many of their needs on grass alone, they are usually the non-lactating cows (i.e., cows that aren't producing milk).

A modern dairy cow consuming grass alone would be equivalent to a marathon runner or Olympic athlete consuming only lettuce with a few sprigs of broccoli. In the old days, everyone had a couple cows, and they only needed to make enough milk for their family. Thanks to genetics and modern management practices, a dairy cow now makes about 10 gallons of milk every day. On grass alone, a modern average producing lactating dairy cow would eventually lose tremendous amounts of weight and be unhealthy. We feed corn and other protein sources to keep them healthy. As a dairy cow nutritionist, I make sure cows have all the needed nutrients to perform and remain healthy while producing healthy nutritious milk.

A typical dairy cow's diet consists of around 50% forage* and 50% grains. Most of the forages are plant material that is fed as hay or fermented forage, known as silage.* This allows farmers to feed grass, legume and corn-based forages year round. The most common concentrates fed are corn and soybeans, along with by-product feeds like whole cottonseeds, citrus pulp, almond hulls or soy hulls. Cows enjoy variety in their diets, and having a mix of both forage and concentrates allows this. Just like with human nutrition, we must provide the correct amounts, balance of nutrients and make it appealing.

Cows are different from humans in that:

1. *Cows have a four compartment stomach with a large fermentation vat. This fermentation vat is known as the rumen. In the rumen, bacteria help to digest the feed. This allows cows to obtain nutrition from feedstuffs that contain cellulose and fibrous material that humans and other animals cannot. This is one reason why cows can consume many by—product feeds.*

2. *Cows are limited in the selection of feed that is offered to them. Nutritionists for-mulate their diet, and it's offered to them in one mixed up casserole, called a total mixed ration or TMR. However, cows can be picky, and they will try to sort through the feed offered to them. Just like humans, they prefer some feedstuffs to others.*

3. *Cows also have the ability to ruminate. They eat their meals rather quickly, and then while resting, they will further digest the feed that was consumed. They regurgitate a ball of feed, known as a cud, and then they chew on that cud. It sounds gross, but this allows them to break up the feed into smaller particles. It also produces saliva, which helps to keep the material in the rumen from becom-ing too acidic and cause indigestion.*

As a cow nutritionist, I do have some advantages that I'm sure dietitians would appre-ciate. I can check diets based on records of what's been consumed, chemically analyze that diet, and modify it accordingly... and my clients (the cows) will usually accept my rec-ommendations. Frankly, cows eat better diets than humans!

There are many similarities and a few key differences between the nutritional demands of a cow and a human, as you can see. Cow nutritionists have a common goal with human dietitians—providing a healthy, balanced diet within a budget for our clients. After all, healthy cows provide a healthy product for you!

You can follow Dr. Rastani, PhD, on Twitter (@cow nutritionist) to learn more about the technical aspects of cow dietetics and all things Packers, especially during Packers football games. You'll also find her with a Spotted Cow during the games (I'll let you figure that one out).

Because I'm married to a ruminant* nutritionist, I can personally attest to the amount of work, science, and time spent on diets for cattle. If you have concerns about what animals are being fed, ask the experts. They use common sense in bal-ancing diets to be sure cows are in the best shape possible to make your food.

Fertilizers, pests and protecting the environment

Do you like to garden? If you do, you likely appreciate the effort it takes to work the soil, ensure the proper amounts of nutrients for plants, and protect the food from pests (weeds, bugs, fungus, and the like). Gardeners can probably relate to the steps a farmer goes through, though the farmer's steps are far more precise than those of most of us who garden.

Remember Darin, the farmer in northeast Kansas? He has the iPad-loving little boy who "farms" in their basement with his toys. Darin explains how he cares for the environment while also protecting the soil, one of his farm's greatest assets:

Before we even think about planting, we start with the soil sample. Using GPS-guided four-wheelers, we pull soil samples across a field to determine nutrient levels. The soil is analyzed at a laboratory, telling us how many nutrients we may need to add for opti-mum crop production.

The big improvement in soil sampling in the last 20-30 years is the move to GPS-based sampling, sampling smaller areas of the field and then using treatments based on

specifically what a given area of the field needs. This keeps us from putting too much fertilizer on an area that already has enough, while preventing runoff and contamination from excess nutrients, as well as putting more nutrients where the crop can really use them.

The next big technological advancement is what we don't do: no-till.* For generations, farmers plowed the soil in preparation for planting. In many areas of the country, no tillage is performed ahead of planting today. This has numerous benefits. It protects the soil much better from wind and water erosion, reduces fossil fuel use, and in drier areas, helps conserve water.

It's one of those less-sexy technologies that's allowed for huge advancements in the environmental sustainability of modern agriculture. Practices and situations vary widely across the country; for example, in the northern areas, technology has simply enabled them to grow crops like corn, and so they have to work the soil in order to warm it up quickly in the spring.

Believe it or not, we begin thinking about next year's corn crop in the fall, which is when we fertilize. We apply nitrogen in the soil in the fall so that as soon as weather and conditions allow in the spring, we can begin corn planting. Nitrogen application is guided by GPS. It's the same set of satellites you would use in your car, but at a much, much higher level of accuracy.

Using on-ground base stations with the satellites, equipment can be steered to accuracy of less than 1 inch. This allows us to practice something we call strip-till, where we are applying nitrogen fertilizer in a strip, tilling the soil in that strip, and then coming back and planting on top of that exact same strip next spring. This is all guided by satellites miles above us. The benefits of strip-till are a better crop seedbed while maintaining the no-till benefits across most of the field.

Finally, we reach the point of planting the crop. The seed we use has been bred using a variety of high-tech methods for maximum resistance to a wide range of diseases and pests. Also, drought tolerance, or the ability of the corn plant to survive periods of water stress during the growing season, is a growing focus.

The planter we use is designed to space seeds uniformly across the entire field. All of this takes an incredible amount of precision engineering. The goal is always the same: allow that seed the best possible chance to germinate, to grow, and to produce a good crop.

There are many different ways to farm, but practices like these are consistently performed across the country regardless of conventional or organic, large or small. Ninety-nine percent (99%) of farmers say they care about environmental practices, while nearly 75% of consumers are concerned about the use of pesticides and insecticides* used in farming.[34] Doesn't it make sense that we talk about the environment?

It's common sense that plants need to be fertilized and protected from many pests, right? Fertilizer is the food for the plant and where there are plants, there are bugs. Hopefully, Darin's description of the technology used to monitor how the products are used offered you one perspective on the positive use of technology in protecting the environment. You can connect with him at @KansFarmer on Twitter.

Pretty green space

Before I'm accused of spinning the issue of fertilizers/chemical use in farming, let me put in terms that most homeowners can relate to: You know that lush green lawn you enjoy? My daughter and I love to go barefooting (her term) in the yard by our house and barn, so we kill weeds, keep nasty bugs away, and fertilize the yard with urea.*

We're careful to apply products by label recommendations to keep little bare feet off the lawn after it's been sprayed, but not as careful as farmers are in their use of products in their fields. Farmers utilize technology for greater accuracy, undergo certification to apply products properly and follow product labels stating for acceptable rates. Quite different than my weed killing spraying technique!

Homeowners go to great lengths to have outdoor spaces without pests. The National Academy of Science points to lawn use as a significant part of what they say is the "pesticide problem." According to the Environmental Protection Agency (EPA), homeowners use 10 times more pesticides per acre than farmers do, although the farmer uses pesticides more widely.[35] Interestingly—the same website page shows that a riding lawnmower pollutes as much in one hour as does driving a typical automobile for 45 miles.

Is it really applying common sense to believe that farmers are spraying chemicals as much as they can? If direct exposure to the chemicals used in your home and on your lawn hasn't damaged you, it stands to reason that products used in food production won't either. I'm not going to claim that every practice or product in farming is perfect, but I can promise that these practices are done and products are used with a foundation of common sense and a whole lot of research.

Michael Pollan, author of *The Omnivore's Dilemma* and *Food Rules* and other books has some great ideas—and an avid following, especially after the movie *Food, Inc.* I agree with many of his points about eating healthier and appreciate his interest in food as a journalist, but take issue with his representation of modern agriculture.

I find Pollan's work to be divisive in the conversation around the food plate. Some of his ideas lack common sense, largely because of a lack of ongoing firsthand experience and because of a seemingly larger budget than most food buyers can afford. Frankly, many of his ideas are insulting to many in agriculture.

Case in point: farmers are not so ignorant that they can't control their own destiny, nor are they controlled by big business—as Pollan claims. Agriculture is not an industrial revolution but rather a technological adopter. **It is not a perfect system; it's one we continue to improve upon just as agriculture has been improved upon since the start of time.**

One of the challenges agriculture faces is that farming and food processing aren't pretty businesses. Rain can create piles of mud and manure on the most pristine operation. Animals can be very dangerous, as can massive pieces of equipment. Idyllic barns no longer best serve animals or farmers, and facilities that are closed to protect animal health seem secretive to the public.

Today's technology makes farms more akin to something out of The Jetsons than Charlotte's Web. Some of our practices look terrible to the untrained eye, even when they're done in the best interest of the land or animal. Hopefully, common sense prevails to answer the question of why such practices might be used so that it becomes more of a question about "why?" rather than an attack or assuming the worse about agriculture. Consider the example of Princess earlier in this chapter the next time you see another nasty video from animal rights activists.

Practices are constantly reviewed in research and federal agencies so they can be improved in the future, moreso today that at any time in the past. **The intense interest in food (and, therefore, farming) offers the opportunity for a more dynamic**

discussion about what we do throughout the food system, Yet that excitement wanes when rotten vegetables are launched across the food plate.

There are *many* different ways to grow food. Hopefully, you've seen that come to life through both firsthand stories from farmers and a human look at agriculture. If you approach the conversation with labels or perceptions of ignorance, greed, or negativity, you will not find hands reaching across the table, because these labels are very personal to farmers and ranchers.

Common sense is perhaps the most important component of the approach presented in *No More Food Fights!* We all could use more of it, I suspect. How are you applying common sense in making your food decisions?

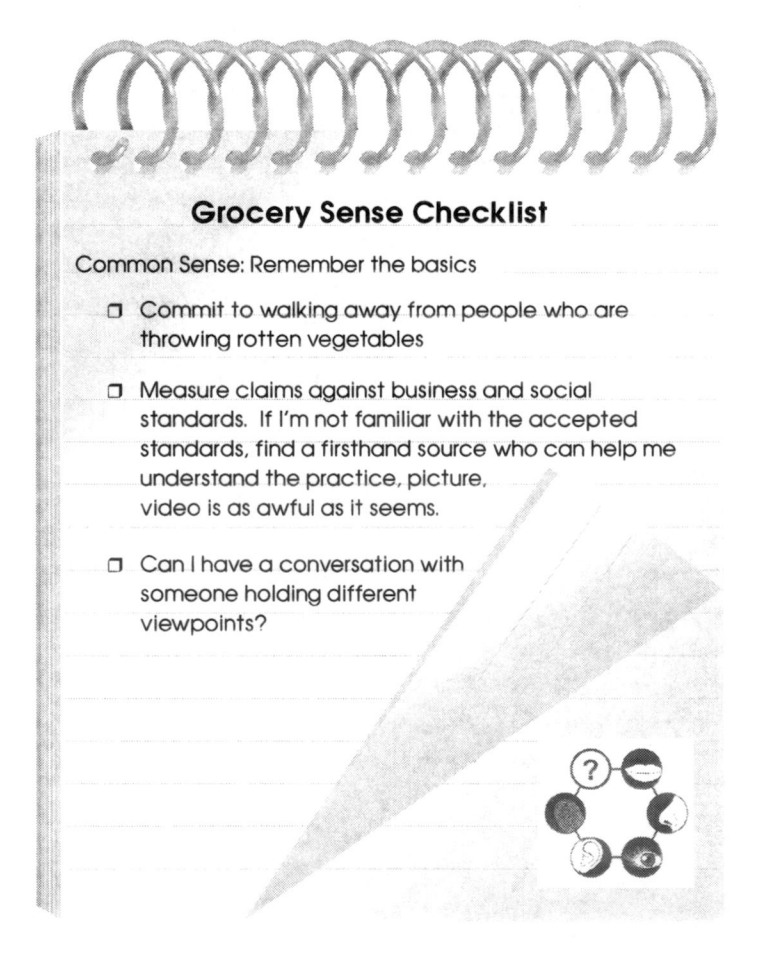

Grocery Sense Checklist

Common Sense: Remember the basics

☐ Commit to walking away from people who are throwing rotten vegetables

☐ Measure claims against business and social standards. If I'm not familiar with the accepted standards, find a firsthand source who can help me understand the practice, picture, video is as awful as it seems.

☐ Can I have a conversation with someone holding different viewpoints?

CHAPTER 7

How Are We Supposed to Talk About Food?

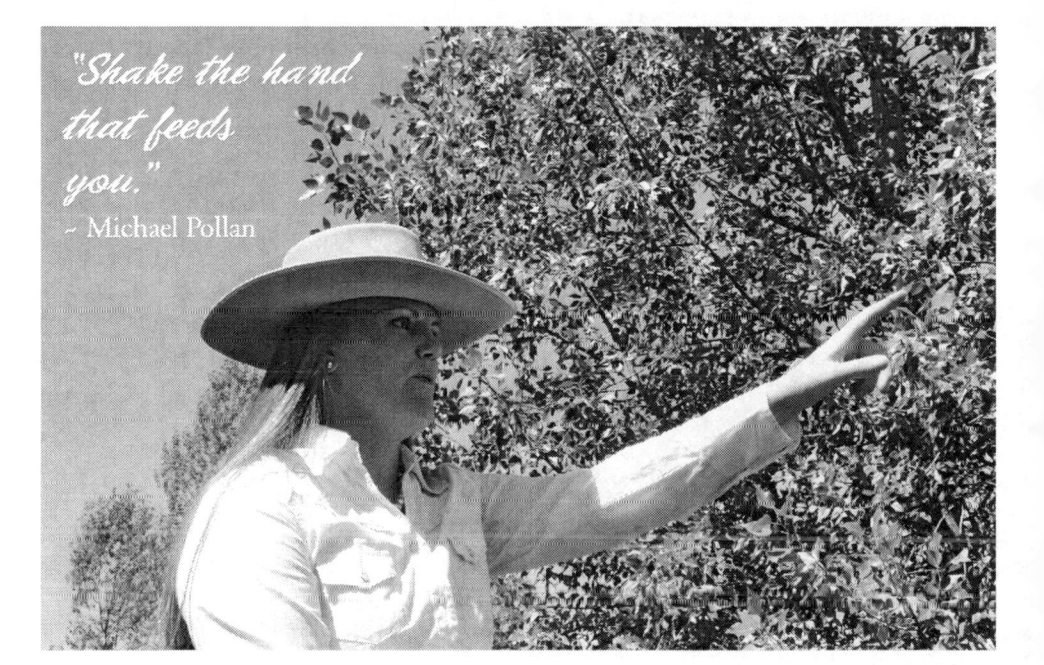

"Shake the hand that feeds you."
- Michael Pollan

"Why do people not care or distrust our role in their food?" asked a group of food microbiologists during lunch in a retro cafeteria at a food industry conference two years ago in Washington, DC. Looking around at the PhD scientists who had dedicated their careers to make food better, I was intrigued and inquired what made the microbiologists think that was the case.

"People don't seem to trust science or want us in their food." There was a lot of truth in that statement, but I suggested the microbiologists spend some time asking questions to clarify people's concerns. In short, they needed to have a conversation with others around the food plate to verify their assumptions.

The hands around the plate represent farmers, dietitians, processors, food scientists, agribusiness, chefs, ranchers, manufacturers, retailers, and more. All are involved in feeding you. My hope is that the six senses will act as a conversation guide so we can do more to reach across the plate to shake those hands.

"The less we know, the more afraid we are likely to be." says David Ropeik in *How Risky Is It, Really?* This book shows that people are more afraid of business and industry, politicians, and processes that are closed and less afraid (more likely to trust)

consumer groups, neutral experts, and processes that are open. So, I have to ask, **how open are we to sharing information from all sides of the food plate to build connections across that plate?**

Garrett Weber-Gale, an Olympic athlete, chef, and owner of food information hub Athletic Foodie™, pointed to the ultimate value in reaching across the plate: "Find multiple sources when you're seeking out information about food. Look for people on the opposite side of the fence, where you'll have a better chance of learning about different sides of the food plate." (You can see more from Garrett and his mission regarding healthy eating in Chapter 6 ½ on the farm side of *No More Food Fights!*)

The reality is that we share common values, but there's a great deal of misinformation driving us apart. Common values must prevail, or we all lose. Food prices will rise, food imports will increase, regulations will drive the system, and misinformation will continue to flourish. I think our food deserves better, don't you? I know our families deserve better.

How can you use these six senses to grow a more meaningful conversation about food?

1. **Touch:** reaching out to farmers
2. **Sight:** clarifying perspective
3. **Sound:** knowing what questions to ask
4. **Smell:** passing the science sniff test
5. **Taste:** feeling good about your personal choice
6. **Common sense:** remembering the basics

Food is an intensely personal choice; no one should dictate the rules for your own plate. Rather, use your senses to find the information to make the right decision for your family. How are you going to do that?

The Grocery Sense Checklists are designed to help you feel good about making food decisions. As Yogi Berra once said "When you come to a fork in the road, take it!" Food is not an 'either-or.' It's a 'both.'

There will be major issues we'll have to agree to disagree on, as you've likely identified while reading *No More Food Fights!* Let's take the fork in the road; agree to disagree on some topics and still shake hands around the food plate on others.

I believe reaching across the food plate can happen if the conversation is approached with curiosity, candor, and civility. After all, we are all humans. We all eat and we all have to buy food. Why not bring some peace to the plate?

Let's meet in the middle. It's much nicer—and smells a lot better—than a food fight.

Grocery Sense Checklist

6 Senses of a meaningful food conversation

- ☐ **Touch:** Have you reached out?
- ☐ **Sight:** Are you clarifying perspective?
- ☐ **Sound:** Can you ask questions?
- ☐ **Smell:** Does information pass the science sniff test?
- ☐ **Taste:** Do you feel good about your choice?.
- ☐ **Common sense:** Have you looked at the basics?

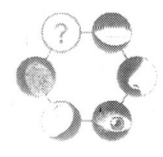

CHAPTER 8

Can You Connect at the Center of the Plate?

"My own experience is to use the tools that are out there. Use the digital world. But never lose sight of the need to reach out and talk to other people who don't share your view.
Listen to them and see if you can find a way to compromise."

~ Colin Powell

Take a look at the plate at the beginning of this chapter. What do you see? A plethora of food? A need for lower food prices? Amazingly diverse products? Nutritional expertise or obesity epidemic ? Brilliant advances or industrial problems? Nutrition for everyone or for only the privileged?

What do you feel when you look at the food plate? Disgust? Hunger? Curious about why your portion of the plate isn't bigger?

ROTTEN VEGETABLE 8
Is your passion driving others away? Are you so outspoken that people only hear you screaming? Passionate agriculture and food people attract others like bees to honey. Sure, some can be passionate naysayers, but it's a small percentage. Why not find common points in your passion to get excited about farming and food together? Hint: this means you have to rein your passion in enough to listen to each other.

Gratitude that the United States and Canada (and most developed countries) have this type of plate available regularly? Confusion about what you're supposed to be doing when you go to the grocery store?

When I look at the plate, I see people with tremendous expertise around all sides of it. Chefs who marry many food flavors, farmers who grow crops and animals, processors who clean and package food, registered dietitians who help us know the best nutrition for our well-being, and many more.

Yet, I also see dividing lines, which frustrates me—as you could tell on the food side of the book with the trip around the grocery store that left me with a headache and a sore tongue. Meat versus vegetables. Dairy versus soy. Small versus large. Organic versus conventional. Corn versus sugar. One label versus another.

The point of *No More Food Fights!* is to encourage a civil conversation; it's about **people working together to understand the many perspectives around the plate.** I'd like to look at that same plate and see polarized conversations move toward the middle.

Compromise can be viewed as a dirty word—some seem to think it means they have to give up their own point of view. Look at it as bringing your own perspective and then adding more ideas to enrich the conversation. The same could be said with meeting in the middle. It's not a political statement in *No More Food Fights!*, but a visual of where we can go to shake hands.

After all, the conversation becomes rather lopsided—and self-serving—causing the plate to go off kilter if it's farm versus food. That's when the food fights begin and can stink up the place. But we can find balance if we meet in the middle.

> **CONNECTION POINT 7**
>
> How do you politely disengage from those not interested in a courteous conversation? My estimate is that 10% on either side of the spectrum (entrenched or inflamed) aren't interested in a lot more than promoting their positions. I suggest that removing the platform from grandstanders takes away their stage, which takes energy from their cause. You do so by thanking them for their time, then walking away—and being disciplined enough to not get into a negative or competitive debate.
>
> Instead, focus on those you can engage in a productive conversation. Productive doesn't equal agreement, but it does equal meaning. Look for common values, human interest, hot buttons. Start there, rather than trying to tackle the major issues first. Each person around the food plate is human, with human interests.

Who can lead the conversation to the center?

"Thought leadership" is a term thrown around a fair amount in the business environment. It may be considered cliché by some or, as I've found, make most people scratch their heads. If you have the ability to approach a subject with perspective on both sides of the issue, you are a thought leader. These are key leadership elements that bridge the gap and bring people to the center of the plate:

- **Passion.** It acts as a magnet. It propels a movement. It engages a community. Thought leaders have the ability to channel their passion for the good of the greater cause.

- **Honesty.** It's easy to pretend to be someone else in today's social media—driven society, and some people thrive on building false profiles. Don't be anyone but you!

- **Ears.** Can you hear a question from across the food plate and really *listen*? Do you automatically go into defense mode? Are you coming up with your answer while the other person is talking? Thought leaders ask others questions and listen closely to the answers.

- **Guts enough to accept change**—and, preferably, embrace it. You're as young as you're ever going to be today—are you really sure you want to spend your life complaining about change? Many reference their ages for not understanding social media, but I've seen 65-year-old grandpas outpace 25-year-old guys in using Facebook. Don't let your birthdate, position, or embarrassment prevent you from adapting to change!

- **Big picture**. Thinking long-term and looking beyond your own business to understand global demands is essential to leading the food and farm conversation. This provides consideration of the impact of policy, activism and markets influencing the big picture conversation.

- **Curiosity.** Children thrive on it; adults bury it. Sometimes, the simple act of asking why can lead you down an entirely different path. Curiosity is an element of leadership that will help you discern what's important to the people you're trying to talk to about food and farm.

- **Execution.** If you don't have the ability to put wheels under ideas and involve others in pulling the wagon, you'll be stuck. Bright shiny objects are fun, but they become dull over time and get put away in the back of the closet. Only those who can execute, stay focused, and grow ideas are true leaders.

- **Open mind.** Many think our greatest days of innovation are in the past. I disagree; the food-and-farm discussion is a frontier desperately in need of thought leadership. Look at the technologies, businesses, communities, and techniques available to you now that didn't exist five years ago. Be open enough to find a way to adapt them for the benefit of the big picture.

- **Tenacity for the long haul.** Few parts of agriculture or food can be called easy business. Agendas around a myriad of issues, often fueled by misinformation, add to the challenge, but always know that one voice, a single picture, or a tweet may just capture the attention of thousands—and make people stop to consider the middle of the plate.

- **Humility** enough to admit when you're wrong and to apologize when needed. There's not a better teacher of this than parenthood. Everyone makes mistakes; own up to them and move on. Humility is rare in those holding leadership positions, but the few who possess it can lead a movement as servant—leaders.

- **Optimism**. If you don't believe in a better tomorrow, why bother?

- **Willingness to have the tough conversations.** Is local and organic better? Do we still need subsidies? Why are your farming/cooking practices better or worse than mine? Do food buyers have a right to demand labels? Are animals

living in better conditions? This is difficult, but thought leadership is about leading the conversation, not reacting to it. It's also about taking the high road even when others sink to the gutter.

Truthfully, I'd like to see more thought leadership in the food and farming conversation. We all sing to the choir that we have to do things differently, so how about we actually put some muscle where our mouths are?

Putting your fork, knife, spoon, and knife to work

Silverware can help with that. Let's take a look at how we can put the fork, spoon, and knife to work in reaching across the plate. Please note: this is reaching—not poking or hitting. Play nice with your silverware.

Fork: Connecting tines

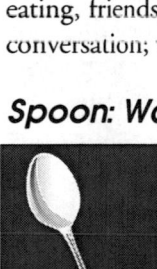

The fork is perhaps the most commonly used utensil in the Western world. It can be used for stabbing, swiping, and scooping food. It can also stick people in the back—as those people who want to throw smelly rotten tomatoes in a food fight seem to do through grandstanding and positioning.

To me, the fork represents a stake in the ground. On one side of the plate, you have the pitchfork. Hopefully you realize by now that modernization has eliminated many pitchforks and farmers don't look like the *American Gothic* farmer portrait, but we're going with a pitchfork as a visual example. These forks are busily at work worrying about what needs to happen on the farm. On the other side, you have the dining fork concerned about feeding a family the best food possible—with conflicting needs depending on socioeconomic status and geography.

Is it possible for those forks to become more similar in their interests? Yes, if both sides pause and look around to see where the commonalities are. After all, we are all humans. Most have an interest in family, sports, school, community, national well-being, eating, friends, and the like. Don't let people around you raise their forks in fear of the conversation; what would happen if the tines connected? A bridge would be formed.

Spoon: Warming the relationship

Pour some sugar on me! Yes, I'm a rock 'n' roll fan, but spoons have such a happy feel to them. Whether you're sipping soup, hanging them from your nose, or eating ice cream, the spoon is a utensil that's not only practical but also warming.

What if we applied that same idea to the conversation around the food plate? I'm not suggesting you spoon with the person you're connecting with around the food plate (bodily spooning would likely create more than food fights!), but I do believe we can easily have a practical discussion. As people find value in the conversation—and an understanding about their particular positions—there will be a warming to the relationship that leads to trust.

Ultimately, that's what brings people to the center of the plate—respect and trust—even when there is not 100% agreement. Remember the spoon to help you warm a relationship.

Knife: Leveraging a community

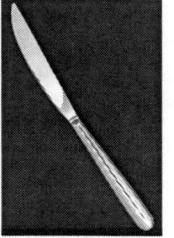

The Transportation Security Administration (TSA) considers the knife a dangerous weapon, and most of you probably have negative images of knives going into skin. Let's look at it in a different light. Imagine this: a few peas placed on the end of the knife, slightly bent back, aimed at the person across the table from you. It's kind of fun to imagine that kind of leveraging, isn't it?

Rather than flinging food, consider the leveraging power knives can have in lifting and moving items. Leveraging is critical in this discussion. Don't just reach your hand across—find others to join you in getting to know people across the table.

In other words, leverage a community to build a movement. After watching thousands of people from around the world connect virtually through communities such as AgChat and FoodChat, I know firsthand the power in building communities that leverage the passions people have about food and farming.

The greatest power we have in this is a combined interest in food and farming. Think of the knife to help you leverage that!

Looking for exact answers in how to have a meaningful conversation? Take a look at the utensils around the plate, and consider how the fork, spoon, and knife can help build connections. Then take a look at the person holding the silverware.

Do you have enough guts to meet in the middle?

True leadership is influence—not only influence within a small circle, but grasping—and in turn influencing—the bigger picture. The conversation around food and farm is in desperate need of those leaders, not of someone who can simply tell his or her story and string a line of manure. Not the most gifted at debate. And certainly not a dictator who sees his or her opinion as the answer for all.

The most effective leaders I've seen combine passion with human-ness, which makes them effective in connecting with others. **Consider the middle of the food plate; it's where hands meet in a handshake, trust is built, and human connections form.**

Thought leadership around the food plate will lead people to the middle—and requires authenticity, a bit of audacity, and a whole lot of action.

Authenticity. Keep it real. What if you were asked to engage in a conversation with 10 people holding different viewpoints about food? It helps to acknowledge that your part of the plate doesn't always get it right, though you try your best.

As discussed throughout this book, neither side of the plate has done the best job at connecting. Don't let food become the next religion and politics—have an open conversation.

Audacity. This is having guts enough to do what needs to be done. To put it in farm terms, will you be the bull or the steer? I'm not suggesting we charge anyone and knock down gates, but perhaps we should be a bit more aggressive in seeking ways to connect—especially in times when there is no war to fight.

In other words, be audacious enough to be proactive—not in a bold, arrogant way, but with enough gumption to try something new, whether it's going beyond the choir or trying out new media.

Action. Are you an active or reactive leader? Leaders don't wait until the rotten veggies are thrown by the other side, because they understand the trust of the middle is being eroded.

Action as a leader in today's hyperconnected world must include the ability to gather and engage the 80% of people who can still be influenced. This action is required in times of response *and* status quo. Meeting in the middle should be a proactive daily occurrence, not a response mechanism.

If you're passionate about any part of the conversation connecting gate to plate, here's my challenge to you: **Authentically consider what you want to accomplish, be audacious enough to try new ideas, and take action to bring others to the table.** In other words, know what your goal is, have the guts to pursue it, and surround yourself with the best people who believe in the cause.

Many have suggested I include screen shots of the grandstanding happening online, examples of conversations gone awry, and specific outlines of what the right kind of conversation looks like in *No More Food Fights!* I'm not doing that because stories interwoven through the 6 ½ steps for the ag folks and the six senses for the food folks are the best examples I can offer.

As I finished writing this book, a great quote from executive coach Scott Eblin popped up in my e-mail: "Keeping people informed keeps them calm."

What is the unique perspective you bring to the table? How are you informing people about your side of the food plate? If each person collectively brings his or her information to the table, I hope we can have the majority of people at the table be calm—and be civil—in our conversation.

Take a look 20 years down the road. What does the food plate look like? Will it be painted by people with authenticity, audacity, and action—or rhetoric? If you think food and farming have changed in the past two decades, be prepared for even greater change—and a greater disconnect.

My single wish? *No More Food Fights!* has made you think about how to grow your conversation about food and farm. You decide who has the vision to make the boldest strokes in reaching across the plate; those will be the people painting the food plate of the future. **I believe we have the opportunity to re-write tomorrow's history of farm and food.**

Actions to connect at the center of the plate are the same whether you're on the farm or food side. If you flip the book over and read the other side, you'll see this final chapter is identical. That's because reaching across the plate to shake hands looks the same, no matter what angle you approach it from. Are you willing to grow that connection into a more meaningful conversation about food and farm?

References

1 "Supermarket Facts: Industry Overview 2012-2011." *Food Marketing Institute.* http://www.fmi.org/research-resources/supermarket-facts

2 Simmons, Jeff. Summary of studies and key data from the International Consumer Attitudes Study. Plenty to Think About. http://plentytothinkabout.org/wp-content/uploads/2011/03/Three-Rights-White-Paper-Revised.pdf

3 U.S. Farmers and Ranchers Alliance Study. *Food Dialogues.* September 2011.www.fooddialogues.com/resources/usfra-national-infographic-9-21-11.jpg

4 Illinois Farm Families Presentation at Illinois Commodity Conference. November 2011.

5 Dillard, John. "The Myth of the Humane Society of the United States." *University of Richmond School of Law Juris Publici.* January 2010. http://jurispublici.richmond.edu/default.php?pageType=2&docId=45329&docIssue=2010-01-25

6 Caroprese, M. "Relationship Between Cortisol Response to Stress and Behavior, Immune Profile, and Production Performance of Dairy Ewes." *Journal of Dairy Science* 93.6 (2010): 2009-2604. http://www.ncbi.nlm.nih.gov/pubmed/20494148

7 Helm, Janet. "Why You Shouldn't Detox Like Demi (Or Eat Like Gwneth)." *NBC News.* October 2010. http://www.msnbc.msn.com/id/38884072/ns/health-womens_health/#.UMjvSb_lXLY

8 Arnot, Charlie. "Sustainability Requires Balance." *Feedstuffs.* April 2008. http://www.feedstuffs.com/ME2/dirmod.asp?sid=&nm=&type=Publishing&mod=Publications::Article&mid=AA01E1C62E954234AA0052ECD5818EF4&tier=4&id=0F8C62AC1D004902A0BE4519D23A0656

9 Valdes, Alisa. "The Lameness of the LA Times Red Meat Story Part 2." *Miss Alisa's Place.* March 2012. http://missalisasplace.com/2012/03/15/the-lameness-of-the-la-times-red-meat-story-part-2/

10 "Press Freedom Index 2011/2012." *Reporters without Borders: For Freedom of Information.* http://en.rsf.org/press-freedom-index-2011-2012,1043.html

11 The Council for Biotechnology Information (CBI). http://www.whybiotech.com/

12 Agriculture Biotechnology: A Lot More than Just GM Crops. *International Service for the Acquisition of Agri-biotech Applications (ISAAA).* August 2010. http://www.isaaa.org/resources/publications/agricultural_biotechnology/download/default.asp

13 "Corn Background." *USDA Economic Research Service.* November 2012. http://www.ers.usda.gov/topics/crops/corn/background.aspx

14 "Labeling of Bioengineered Foods." *Report 2 of the Council on Science and Public Health.* June 2012. www.ama-assn.org/resources/doc/csaph/a12-csaph2-bioengineeredfoods.pdf

[15] Ropeik, David. *How Risky Is It, Really?* McGraw-Hill, 2012. http://www.dropeik.com/how_excerpt.html

[16] Kotecki, Jason. *The Official Adultitis website.* http://www.adultitis.org/

[17] "Milk Marketing Order Statistics: Retail Milk Prices." *USDA Agricultural Marketing Service.* March 2012. http://www.ams.usda.gov/AMSv1.0/ams.fetchTemplateData.do?template=TemplateL&navID=IndustryMarketingandPromotion&leftNav=IndustryMarketingandPromotion&page=RetailPrices&description=Milk+Marketing+Order+Statistics&acct=dmktord

[18] Vicini, J., et al. "Survey of Retail Milk Composition as Affected by Label Claims Regarding Farm-Management Practices." *Journal of the American Dietetic Association.* 2008:1198-1203.

[19] Walker, G.P., et al. "Effects of Nutrition and Management on the Production of Milk Fat and Protein: A Review." *Australian Journal of Agricultural Research.* 2004: 1009-1028.

[20] Vicini, J., et al. "Survey of Retail Milk Composition as Affected by Label Claims Regarding Farm-Management Practices." *Journal of the American Dietetic Association.* 2008: 1198-1203.

[21] "National Organic Program." *USDA: Agriculture Marketing Service.* http://www.ams.usda.gov/AMSv1.0/nop

[22] "Kenneth A. Cook: Biography." *Activist Cash.* http://activistcash.com/biography.cfm/b/2825-kenneth-a-cook

[23] Henderson, Greg. "We'll All Be Vegetarians by 2050, Scientists Say." *Drovers Cattle Network.* August 2012. http://www.cattlenetwork.com/e-newsletters/drovers-daily/167746295.html

[24] American Society of Animal Science Board of Directors. "Should the World Go Vegetarian? Scientists Say 'No'." *Drovers Cattle Network.* September 2012. http://www.cattlenetwork.com/e-newsletters/drovers-daily/Should-the-world-go-vegetarian-Scientists-say-no-168183726.html

[25] Bodnar, Anastasia, @geneticmaize. *Twitter.* September 2012. https://twitter.com/geneticmaize/status/244421919322013696

[26] Kaye, Leon. "Is America beyond Peak Meat?" *Triple Pundit: People, Planet, Profit.* March 2012. http://www.triplepundit.com/2012/03/meat-consumption-united-states/

[27] "Food Consumption & Demand." *USDA.* July 2012. http://www.ers.usda.gov/topics/food-choices-health/food-consumption-demand.aspx

[28] Bottemiller, Helena. "Confidence in Food Safety Slipping, Industry Survey Finds." *Food Safety News.* October 2011. http://www.foodsafetynews.com/2011/10/confidence-in-food-safety-slipping-industry-survey-finds/#.UMoAsXPjlWY

[29] Webster, Maeve. "Perception versus Reality: A Food Study." *Charleston | Orwig.* http://charlestonorwig.com/2012Event/perception.aspx

[30] "Hunger Stats." *World Food Programme.* http://www.wfp.org/hunger/stats

[31] Simmons, Jeff. "Making Safe, Affordable and Abundant Food a Global Reality." *Plenty to Think About.* March 2011. http://plentytothinkabout.org/wp-content/uploads/2011/03/Three-Rights-White-Paper-Revised.pdf

[32] Desrochers, Pierre and Hiroko Shimizu. *The Locavore's Dilemma: In Praise of the 10,000-mile Diet.* PublicAffairs, 2012.

[33] Bailey, Ronald. Editorial reviews The Locavore's Dilemma: In Praise of the 10,000-mile Diet. *Amazon.com.* http://www.amazon.com/The-Locavores-Dilemma-Praise-000-mile/dp/1586489402

[34] "US Farmers and Ranchers Alliance National Infographic." *Food Dialogues.* September 2011. http://www.fooddialogues.com/resources/usfra-national-infographic-9-21-11.jpg

[35] Aagesen, Colleen and Mary Fiscus. "Can Lawns Kill?" *EPA Green Landscaping: Greenacres.* November 2012. http://www.epa.gov/greenacres/wildones/handbk/wo8.html#Can%20Lawns

Glossary of Terms

*W*elcome to my non-technical explanation of agricultural terms and practices used by farmers in this book. Rather than providing the science and technical jargon to define these agricultural terms, this is my translation of farm language to the rest of the world. I've tried to explain them in a way that relates to the majority of the population. There are thousands of terms to define, so this list only includes * terms used in No More Food Fights!

Biotechnology: Taking one gene (a small part of DNA) from one plant and placing it in another. Think seedless watermelons and grapes. Contrary to rumors, approved biotechnology uses naturally occurring genes and is heavily researched. For example, companies invest around $150 million and 15 years in research before biotechnology seeds are approved—far more than any "regular" seed. Biotechnology was named genetically engineered and genetically modified organisms by activists interested in fear mongering when it was first approved by USDA.

Boluses: Large pills given to large animals through a tube that protects their throat and human hands. Boluses are given when medication is needed to help an animal feel better (e.g. aspirin or a massive dose of vitamins) or as a preventative (e.g. giving a heifer a magnet to protect her stomach from a metal object she might eat).

Conventional: Common term for modern farming practices, but also used to describe a farm that is not certified organic. Conventional farms can be small or large. Conventional practices can include no-till and GPS. These farms adapt a wide variety of practices and technologies. Some are grass fed, others farm thousands of acres. Just as schools have too many labels today, so do farms. I think of a farmer as a farmer, regardless of the label.

Cow tipping: A myth about being able to tip cows over while they're sleeping. Cows lay down while sleeping, so this particular myth annoys me. Besides, cows are way too smart to let a strange human come up and "tip" them without extending their rear foot in greeting.

Crop rotation: The practice of rotating the different kinds of crops (seeds) planted each year to protect the soil, reduce disease and maximize productivity. Know how you're not supposed to plant tomatoes in the same are of your garden year after year? The same applies to a farmer's fields.

European Corn Borer: As you might expect from the name, this insect bores into the plant and ear of corn. In addition to damaging the ear of corn, it weakens the plant and leaves it susceptible to disease and weather damage. Plants have been bred to be resistant to this one virulent pest.

Forage: Roughage, such as alfalfa, corn, oats, wheat or sorghum that provide fiber and starch in an animal's diet. Either chopped into small pieces to become silage or baled. You could also draw a comparison with multi-grain bread or breakfast cereal.

Free stall: An individual bed for animals to keep them clean and comfortable. Their bedding may be sand, sawdust, recycled materials or a waterbed mattress. Free stalls are typically metal u-shaped tubes so the animals (most commonly dairy cows) have an area where other animals don't injure them. If you ever had another cow step on your teats, you'd understand. Free stalls usually are "laundered" a few times a week at minimum since cows don't use toilets.

GPS-assisted swath control: You know you can adjust your fertilizer spreader to put more or less product on your lawn? The same is true for fields, except the term for how far the product spreads is "swath". Swath control on farms uses a GPS system to understand the areas of the field that have already had a product (fertilizer for example) applied and automatically shuts portions of the application equipment off to only apply product exactly where it is needed. It's better for the environment and saves money, too.

Haymow: The area where hay (also known as forage, alfalfa or grass) is stored to keep it out of the elements. Historically, the haymow was most commonly found on the second floor of a barn. Today's large bales are typically stored in their own barn to be sure they offer the best nutrition possible for animals.

Heifer: A female bovine (beef or dairy animal) that has not given birth. Heifers usually calve around two years old to be sure they are grown and ready to give milk. This is another term to refrain from using when describing humans.

High Fructose Corn Syrup (HFCS): Take a look at the Karo in your pantry or at a grocery store. It's a sweetener that was likely used by your great grandmother; it has been common in home kitchens for decades. HFCS has come under firestorm for the commercial use of it as a sweetener. It's a by-product of wet milling corn and meets the FDA requirements for the use of the term 'natural.' Personally, I think the discussion about the role of HFCS in the obesity debate would do better to center on people balancing calorie intake with exercise.

Humus: Organic matter found in the soil, not the yummy treat in your refrigerator (hummus). Think happy earthworms—they love humus, which is partially decayed plant or animal matter to provide nutrients for plants and helps the soil stay moist. Black soil has a lot of humus.

Irrigation pumps: This is similar to your lawn sprinkler, but on a much larger scale. An irrigation pump moves the large volumes of water used in irrigation from either an underground source (well) or an above ground source like a pond or creek to the irrigation unit in the field that waters the crop.

Moisture | Temperature sensors in bin: Have you ever had your sugar get nasty from not being stored properly? Same is true for grains, only they're stored in large metal bins. Placing sensors in a grain bin allows a farmer to monitor the quality of the grain. The moisture sensors allow the grain to be dried to the proper level. The temperature sensors alert to any problems with grain quality, as grain that is at risk of declining quality will show rising temperatures. I wish I had that for my sugar bowl!

No-till: A modern farming practice that conserves both topsoil and water. Rather than tilling the soil in the spring, farmers will plant seeds without working the land first and then apply herbicide for weed control. Colder states are not favorable to no-till, as turning over the soil allows it to warm faster (making it ready to be planted) in the spring.

Organic: The USDA Organic label is the only certified federal program, so look for that seal if you want organics. USDA defines organic as "a labeling term that indicates that the food or other agricultural product has been produced through approved methods that integrate cultural, biological, and mechanical practices that foster cycling of resources, promote ecological balance, and conserve biodiversity. Synthetic fertilizers, sewage sludge, irradiation, and genetic engineering may not be used." Please note that this does not mean that pesticides, insecticides, fungicides and fertilizers are not used. You can find USDA organic regulations at http://foodconvo.com/X5LDpE and Canadian regulations at http://foodconvo.com/ZlCyyy.

Pesticides | Insecticides | Fungicides: Products used to kill or stop insects, rodents or fungi. Weed killer, ant spray and athlete's foot treatment are household examples of these products. These can be naturally occurring or man-made. The use of pesticides, insecticides and fungicides in both organic and conventional farming is heavily regulated. Farmers are required to attend training in safe handling, application and disposal of these products. Most farmers use the products sparingly to protect their land, animals, water and families—as well as keep costs down. If you've ever grown a garden, you know there will be bugs of some sort to manage where there are plants and animals.

Plowing | Disking | Ripping: This does not have to do with snow in your driveway or a DJ. These are all different ways of turning over soil in a field. Farm practices vary across the country, but the soil is worked in the spring before planting or following harvest to reduce compaction, help prepare a seedbed and till in organic matter. Think of a roto-tiller for your yard and garden, but on a much larger scale.

Precision controlled seed placement: Can you tell exactly where you planted a flower? This recently developed tool allows farmers to monitor exactly where their seed is going. This helps them grow a uniform, even "stand" (crop) that is most likely to be healthy and have the best yield.

Ruminant: Animals such as cattle, sheep, buffalo and goats have a unique stomach that is divided into four compartments that serve a different function. These can also be described as four stomachs, but it is actually divided in to different "rooms" called the rumen, reticulum, omasum and abomasum. Ruminants can convert otherwise unusable plant materials into nutritious food and fiber, which makes them great recyclers, turning grass and feed into meat and milk. If you had four compartments like a ruminant, you'd enjoy regurgitating your food and chewing your cud, too.

Silage: Fermented, chopped up feed, which ruminants love. Think of hops fermented into beer for a human example, though cows aren't getting drunk off of their silage. It's a base ingredient in most diets for ruminants. Types include haylage, corn silage, oatlage, etc.

Soil erosion: Soil is a farm's greatest asset; many technologies and farming practices are focused on protecting soil. Wind and water are the greatest causes of eroding soil. Think about sand dunes eroding; it's about the same concept in fields.

Soil testing: Samples of soil, usually plugs, are taken from various parts of a field to analyze the soil content and/or needs in a laboratory. Like a blood sample, a soil sample can tell a whole lot about the health of the soil.

Steer: A male bovine (beef or dairy animal) that has been castrated. This is done for safety, food quality and efficiency reasons. Castrated animals are much safer to handle, as bulls can be pretty mean—even without seeing anything red.

Sustainability: This term is thrown around the food plate so much that it could be a hot potato! There are many definitions, but I believe the true sustainability includes environmental, economic and community meanings. Consider your favorite local business. Will it be around long-term if they don't take care of the environment, lack the income to sustain the business and fail to contribute to the community in a meaningful way? Likely not. The same is true on farms and ranches.

Urea: While also produced in your liver during the breakdown of protein, this refers to Urea used in agriculture. Urea contains 46% nitrogen, making it great fertilizer to feed plants such as corn, your lawn and other crops.

Yield monitor on the combine: This nifty tool allows a farmer to instantly see the yield while combining (harvesting) a field. When combined with a GPS device, it allows the data to be recorded along with location information that can produce a map showing how each area of the field yielded. It's kind of like mapping out a report card for a field to see how well it produced.

About the Author

A farm girl since birth and a foodie since eating in Italy, Michele Payn-Knoper is one of North America's leading farm and food advocates. She has helped thousands of people in agricultural, dietetic, and food audiences connect the farm gate to the food plate.

Michele wrote *No More Food Fights!* to encourage people around the food plate to connect in the interest of growing a more productive conversation. After all, food fights can be fun, but they usually end up stinking! She invites you to explore the different sides of the plate and to think about food a little differently as you make decisions for your family.

Michele has built farm and food connections in more than 25 countries and earned the Certified Speaking Professional designation awarded to less than 10% of professional speakers globally. She also founded AgChat and FoodChat, virtual communities connecting thousands of agriculture and food people—many of whom are featured in *No More Food Fights!* Michele is an in-demand media resource whose work has been featured across agricultural media, on food panels, and in major media channels such as *USA Today* and *CNN* to translate firsthand farm experience to the 98.5% of the population not on a farm.

She has owned cattle and baked bread since she was nine years old, and she believes her life's calling is to connect those two worlds. Michele provides a framework for farmers, dietitians, chefs, food scientists, ranchers, consumers, agribusiness, and foodies to reach across the plate and shake hands. She holds BS degrees in animal science and agricultural communications from Michigan State University, where the story of her impact has been featured in a *Spartan Saga*.

Widely recognized for the passion and fire she brings to agriculture and nutrition organizations across the United States and Canada, Michele knows her best audience is in her family's kitchen and barn in west central Indiana. That's where food—and conversation—is to be appreciated, enjoyed, and even celebrated. She invites others to join her in the journey toward connecting farm and food.

MPK Wants to Hear From You!

Want to arrange for Michele to help your group grow the conversation around food and agriculture? Discover for yourself why she's known for lighting up a room, taking audiences on a roller coaster of emotions—and getting them kickboxing. Visit http://causematters.com for MPK's speaking programs and for her *Gate to Plate* blog.

Looking for connections happening around the food plate right now? Interested in resources for the international agriculture and dietetic communities? Check out MPK's Facebook page at http://facebook.com/causematters or follow @mpaynknoper on Twitter at http://twitter.com/mpaynknoper.

Ready to share a story about how you've seen growth in the farm-and-food conversation? Have a great example of people reaching across the plate? With your permission, Michele may feature your work as an example. E-mail your story to book@causematters.com.

In the meantime, keep reaching across the plate!

Use this QR code for
extras to help you
grow the conversation